HI,
ANXIETY

LIFE WITH A
BAD CASE
OF NERVES

KAT KINSMAN

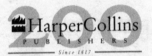

HarperCollins books may be purchased for educational, business, or sales promotional use. For information, please e-mail the Special Markets Department at SPsales@harpercollins.com.

A hardcover edition of this book was published in 2016 by Dey Street Books, an imprint of William Morrow Publishers.

FIRST DEY STREET BOOKS PAPERBACK EDITION PUBLISHED 2017.

Designed by Paula Russell Szafranski

Library of Congress Cataloging-in-Publication Data

Names: Kinsman, Kat, 1972–
Title: Hi, anxiety : life with a bad case of nerves / Kat Kinsman.
Description: First edition. | New York, NY : Dey Street, 2016.
Identifiers: LCCN 2016030635 (print) | LCCN 2016040153 (ebook) | ISBN
    9780062369680 (hardcover) | ISBN 9780062369697 (trade pb) | ISBN
    9780062643278 (audio) | ISBN 9780062369703 (E-Book)
Subjects: LCSH: Depression, Mental—Popular works. | Depression,
    Mental—Treatment—Popular works. | Anxiety in women—Popular works. |
    Women—Psychology—Popular works.
Classification: LCC RC537 .K5345 2016 (print) | LCC RC537 (ebook) | DDC
    616.85/270092 [B]—dc23

978-0-06-236969-7 (pbk.)

19 20 21   RS/LSC   10 9 8 7 6 5 4 3 2

For Douglas, my favorite of all the people

CONTENTS

Introduction: Opening Scene   1

Chapter One: Naming the Beast   9

IRRATIONAL FEAR #1   **HAVING NO WAY OUT**   17

Chapter Two: All in the Family   23

Chapter Three: School Days   31

IRRATIONAL FEAR #2   **DANCING**   41

Chapter Four: The Number of the Beast   47

Chapter Five: The Horrors of Love   53

IRRATIONAL FEAR #3   **SEEING THE DOCTOR**   79

Chapter Six: In the Dungeon   87

IRRATIONAL FEAR #4   **TALKING ON THE TELEPHONE**   99

Chapter Seven: Drifting, Falling, Landing   103

IRRATIONAL FEAR #5   **GETTING MY HAIR CUT**   119

Chapter Eight: Drugging the Beast   **123**

IRRATIONAL FEAR #6   **HAVING CHILDREN**   **141**

IRRATIONAL FEAR #7   **ALTERNATIVE REMEDIES**   **147**

Chapter Nine: Home Is Where the Fear Hides   **155**

IRRATIONAL FEAR #8   **PICKING THINGS UP**   **177**

Chapter 10: On Money and Futons   **183**

IRRATIONAL FEAR #9   **DRIVING**   **203**

IRRATIONAL FEAR #10   **BEING DRIVEN**   **207**

Closing Scene   **211**

Acknowledgments   **219**

HI, ANXIETY

INTRODUCTION

OPENING SCENE

The house has me in its jaws, and it's not letting go. Cabs aren't quick and planes don't wait, and I have to leave now . . . NOW . . . five minutes ago . . . ten, actually. But I can't. This thing is sinking its teeth into my hem, my skin. In my mind I've started to yowl like an animal snapped in steel jaws.

What's worse is that my husband is standing there, watching me rip apart. I can't stop myself and he can't help me and now I've failed the two of us. "You have to go," he's saying to me, kindly, but that's not what I'm hearing through the thrum of blood in my ears. What I'm hearing is: Go. Because you don't deserve any of this—the warm, safe home, the kind, handsome, hilarious husband and throng of sweet, sleepy dogs who have gathered to see you off—because you can't even manage to take care of the basic things you've been trusted with. Not your work, not your purse, not your keys, not your wedding ring. And certainly not your dignity.

The last time I saw my wedding ring was sometime before 3 A.M. when I finally shut the laptop I'd been bent around for hours, scrambling to finish up some work before I went out of town, lest anyone be disappointed or have their lives made slightly inconvenient in

1

my absence. Stupid, careless me, I should have skipped going out to dinner to get all my work finished. I didn't deserve that bit of social life. I should have stayed home and packed, but I didn't do that either, and after two fitful hours in bed, it was time to sling some clothes in my suitcase and fling myself toward the airport. Only that never happens easily. Why did I think it would be any different this time?

The mass began to form as I stood in front of the bathroom mirror, doing my damnedest to mask the ravages of a sleepless night. Mary Kay, Bobbi Brown, and Max Factor themselves could have manifested fully armed in my Brooklyn bathroom, taken one look at my pillow-creased, black-eyed face, and they'd have fled. But there I am, eyeliner wand in fist, attempting to make myself look like a member of the human race when the worry starts thickening in my core. My panic shifts shape each time it appears: sometimes a fist clutched around my windpipe, a grotesquely flexed jaw eroding my molars molecule by molecule, neck and back needled in electric tension, guts dissolving into liquid or a ratatat heartbeat that shocks me out of sleep and leaves me there, awake, no matter how rude the hour.

This particular morning, heat is leaching from somewhere between my shoulder blades, prickling up sweat beads in its path down my back, up to my cheeks, and out to my fingers, which were doing an even piss-poorer job than usual at sketching the edges of my eyelid. Whoops—a sudden bobble of my hand lands the wand on the bathroom floor and a kohl-black waterproof smudge on the bridge of my nose. I shake when I'm nervous, drop things and fumble the pickup. I pull the unzipped suitcase off the bed (promptly dumping the contents onto the bedroom carpet) then stumble over my sweet little wraith of a whippet on the way down the stairs. I bark my annoyance at her and am instantly flooded with shame. She's ancient and fading and I have gotten it in my head lately that she's going to slip away while I'm out of town and (1.) I won't be there to hold her and (2.) the last thing that she'll remember about me was that I was unkind to her. I bend down, memorizing the silken curve of her neck with my hands for the millionth time. It stills them for a moment.

But while patient dogs wait—the world (or at least the TSA) is not possessed of such mercy, and I am not about to let down the people who have paid for my travel if I miss my flight. I heave the jumble-stuffed suitcase to the front door and turn around to scrape my rings from the mantel to my fingers. Only they aren't all there. My right-hand ring and engagement ring are present and accounted for, but my wedding band has vanished.

I sink to the floor, patting around desperately on the carpet in the predawn light because it must be there itmustitmustitmust but it isn't, and as I stand the edges of my vision begin to dissolve into gray. I draw together the last scraps of sanity and breath I have and walk to the landing to call upstairs to my husband. I try to sound as calm as possible, no mean feat, as I don't want to scare the hell out of him.

"Darling, um, could you please come down here for a moment? I am melting down."

Douglas, among his many wonderful qualities, tends to be unflappable in the face of my madness, and an early riser to boot—I'm not yet so far gone that I'd rouse him from his sleep to deal with a lost object crisis—so I knew he'd be awake. Moments later, he clatters downstairs, takes one look at my strained, stained face, and lacquers on some preventive cheer. "What can I help you with, baby?"

I manage, through a series of gestures and noises, to convey to him that I am down a ring, the important one, I hope he doesn't take it to mean that I don't believe in our marriage and treasure our bond, and though I am clearly incompetent, irresponsible, and unworthy of adult, romantic love, would he please not stop giving that love to me, and could he please get down on the carpet—or at least hold the dogs out of the way—and help me locate this sacred symbol of our union in which I obviously do not deserve to be.

After a few, futile minutes, he pulls me back up. "We are not going to find it right now, but I will when I do some housecleaning this weekend. But you have to get on the road now." I nod, gasping for air, sorry for him that he has to be tethered to me. Perhaps while I am away, and our whippet is dying, he'll decide that the ring had the right idea, but meanwhile, he is escorting me to the door, handing me my shoulder bag and the handle of my suitcase while the dogs sidle over to check if they are expected to leave the house at this hour, too. I loop my purse around my other shoulder and the motion seems to jog Douglas's memory.

"Oh, do you have the car key? I need to move it later."

I freeze. In a laughably optimistic attempt to pretend that I could ever live life as anything other than a messy, adolescent horror show, I'd recently bought a royal-blue leather purse (on sale, because retail is for people who can be trusted with nice things) small enough to allow only the essentials of grown-up-lady life: house and office keys, phone, ID, credit cards, lipstick, a thumb drive (or two, or five), a pen, and a small notebook. And that had worked well for all of a week or so before the cursed thing was jammed with receipts, loose change, wrappers, random business cards, mail, and right this minute, the keys to the car. I'd borrowed them briefly to retrieve something from the glove box the day before and they'd been swallowed whole into the garbage pit that is my purse. I begin to dig, spilling dollar bills, my license, insurance card, MetroCard (what's this "wallet" of which you organized people speak?) on the floor while the chaos and worry ferment and swell.

"Baby, it's okay. I'll use the other set. But you have to go."

I go, all right, but not anywhere good. I hear myself scream, and feel the blazing trail of pain it's scratched on its way from my lungs to my throat. Oh God. It's happening and I cannot tamp it down. I've seen this before, my mother contorted, bellowing, her anxiety taking the shape of shrieks, aches, medicine bottles, missed flights, and hospital windows. I'm still fumbling for the car key because I will find it and show it to Douglas and he will know I'm still worth loving.

"Please don't give up on me."

"Baby, you have to leave."

"Don't stop loving me. Please . . . please." I close my fingers around the thick fob and thrust it out to him, sobbing. It is proof that there is some sanity left. I make him hold me for a moment, and he's ginger about it—or so I tell myself. Ten years together and I've wrecked it all by letting him see that I'm helpless against my own head, hands, and mind.

I haul my suitcase down the concrete step to the sidewalk and the wheels rumble behind me down the hill. The sun isn't quite up yet, and I am utterly, completely exhausted.

At the car-service office, I slide into the back of an ancient town car, mutter, "LaGuardia, please," and start tapping out messages.

I'm sorry. Send.

Please don't stop loving me. Send.

There is no response. I fumble for one of the several billion wadded-up tissues in my bag and my fingertips brush against a familiar surface. I pull it out, a custom-made Plexiglas necklace in the form of the word "anxious" with a small lightning bolt swinging from it—and something else. Goddammitwhatthehellohhowironicandstupid.

And thank goodness, the ring is in a pocket in my purse. Send.

His reply is swift. *I love you very much! Glad you found the ring. Just keep breathing and now go and enjoy ATL.*

My brain and eyeballs are pounding. My throat is scorched from chest to tonsils in the wake of my screams, but even so, I begin to relax the tiniest bit. I'm not actually afraid of flying—just getting to the airport (and out of the house). But the northbound traffic on the Brooklyn–Queens Expressway is moving at a decent clip for this hour and I might actually make it there in time for a preflight egg sandwich.

That is, up until the jackknifed tractor-trailer, stretched across all three lanes of traffic on the southbound side, the half-flattened SUV up against the far guardrail, and the swarm of halt-stopped cars maddened, alive and mounting behind them by the second.

I reflexively mumble a quick prayer and crane my neck, looking backward to see if anyone emerges from the smashed car.

No one could have seen this coming. A jumbo-jet-ful of preemptive fretting could not have stopped that accident from happening. It just did. Did they kiss their spouse, their kids, their sweet old dog before they left home, let them know they were loved before they said good-bye? Perhaps, perhaps not. And that worries me, too.

Did your throat close up just a little bit reading this? Spine prickle and tighten, stomach twitch, or did you feel the sweat pooling at the small of your back because it sounded painfully familiar? You're not alone. There are millions of us struggling to fight anxiety in all its forms, every waking (and sometimes sleeping) hour of every day, and we're suffering silently because we don't want to be judged or add to anyone else's burden.

Take my hand. I hope you don't mind if it's shaking a little. We'll get through this together.

These are my stories and thoughts on life with anxiety—but just to be clear, many of the names contained herein are changed. They should not have to worry that anyone will find out their secrets.

CHAPTER ONE

Naming the Beast

When you're too small and tender to know all that much about who you're going to be, the people around you are more than happy to fill in the blanks.

Sometimes this assessment is objective: "Brianna, you are going to be a heartbreaker! And so tall! Have they grabbed you for the basketball team yet?" "Tyler, I heard you won that Math Bowl. Headed for MIT?"

Sometimes, it's evaluative: "Gwen, you've got such a pretty face, but if you don't slim down a little, no boys will ever ask you to dance." "Listen, if you don't take your nose out of that book and get some fresh air and some sun on that pasty skin, you're never going to grow up big and strong like your brother."

Rarely is it helpful—or accurate or binding, for that matter. But when it's couched in concern or love from people who have an interest in the outcome, you tend to believe them and adjust accordingly if possible.

I couldn't.

I can't.

At times—not all the time but often, my hands quiver, my lungs catch, and my stomach stings. It has been that way as long as I recall, is now at the moment I am writing these words, and ever shall be, unless modern medicine develops a pill that doesn't make my metabolism crawl and my brain shock and spit like a downed power line. (I'm not holding my breath.)

Worry and its physical manifestations are part of who I am, from soul to skin. They're an invisible strand twisted tightly into my DNA, mapping its mark on my body in hard scars I cannot stop clawing, the ragged tang of chewed-up cheek flesh, and the slump of my shoulders after another restless attempt at sleep.

My shadow twin didn't have a name at birth, but my teachers and classmates gave it one:

Nervous.

It could have been worse, as I learned when we reached school age. One boy, Jack, was tagged with "Spazzy" (looking back, it seems awfully apparent that he buzzed somewhere deep along the autism spectrum and wasn't receiving any sort of help that I knew of) and was shunned for fear that he'd lash out and hit.

But none of them ever sat quite right on my frame. I was ugly, sure, with an outsized nose and a raggedy, home-trimmed attempt at a Dorothy Hamill haircut, but having my neighbor Robbie as my best friend made me an honorary boy, so that didn't matter all that much. I played sports with great enthusiasm but little endurance or skill, so I wasn't a jock. The appeal of dolls and playing house eluded me, and if forced into a role, I'd assign myself family dog (who was mysteriously able to read), so I could hunch under the table with a book, occasionally whimpering and wagging out of bored commitment to the task.

Mainly, and I still feel shy about stating it, I was the smart girl. In our enlightened, electronically amplified times, celebrities and activists take to the virtual airwaves touting the badassery and supremacy of academically inclined young ladies: smart girls rule and/or rock! Smart is the new pretty! Everyone likes the smart girl at the party!

It's empowering and laudable, but back then, little would have mortified me more. Books, paper, and pencils were my refuge in a world where I already knew that pretty was a currency I lacked, *and* that my home life was something I suspected was outside the norm. To share my smarts, my difference, with the world was the last thing in the world I wanted.

I wasn't given an option.

The teachers at Ruth Moyer Public Kindergarten weren't fooling a single soul by herding us into animal-themed groups after our first reading test. Kids can sniff a hierarchy at a hundred paces, and as one of only two girls in the "Giraffe" group, I could feel the narrowed eyes of Elle and her pride in the "Tiger" pen, boring into the length of my neck, waiting for us to stumble.

Elle's older sister, who was in my older sister's grade, had given her the lay of the land, and a mandate to knock down anyone who stood out. "Those Kinsman girls think they're better than us. Make sure yours knows she's not."

As it happened, my sister and I were under no such impression—we just happened to be towed to a town where most families had laid down roots many decades back, by parents who'd never met a bit of Victorian literature they didn't like. We read. It wasn't optional in our house, but it wasn't an obligation either. An obligation would have been fine by me.

On that first read-aloud day, when our small groups were loosed from our pens, we hunkered down in a doubled half-moon on the floor around our teacher. One by one, we were called on to stand up and read through the lesson as best we could. I'd galloped through my recitation as I practiced alongside my fellow Giraffes, but as my turn to read in front of the whole class drew near, my breath grew short. I was going to pay for it and I knew it, but I just couldn't dishonor the words by fumbling them.

The teacher called my name and the force of it yanked me to my feet. "Um . . . okay . . . I . . ."

"Hey, what's wrong with Katie's hands?" Before I could get the first words past my bitten lips, Elle's whisper set off a wave of titters that lapped over my skin like an acid bath. I looked down and there was definitely something . . . odd going on.

It was as if my fingers had suddenly declared complete independence from the rest of my appendages. Rather than performing the job they were meant to do—holding my textbook still so I could muscle through the assignment—they'd decided to take on the task of flapping and flying me off to somewhere vaguely less mortifying. A-plus for initiative, hands, but an F on the practicality front, because I could barely make out the words on the page shaking in front of me.

The instructor wasn't granting me safe passage either. She was a no-nonsense schoolmistress with little patience for variation from the formula she'd been using to churn out compliant kindergarteners for the past thirty . . . forty . . . one hundred years. She'd already made it clear to me in the first few weeks of school that she had no interest in spending any extra time on students who wouldn't or couldn't mold their contours to her liking.

"KATIE! Stop being so nervous! You're holding everyone up!" she boomed, shocking me into motion. Suddenly there was a word for the feeling that sometimes clenched my body in its fist and shook it to the point of near explosion.

For reasons that I still can't explain, I inhaled a shuddering breath and huffed out my section of the text in a bizarre Pepé Le Pew accent before folding my knocking knees back together and plopping to the floor. (I have no earthly idea—I just watched a lot of Saturday-morning TV, and I suppose my weirdo kid brain had processed the cartoon skunk as "confident" and "sophisticated.")

This strange performance earned me a brief titter from the class before the next student rose up to muscle through his passage.

Later, during nap time, with all eyes off me, I stretched out uncharacteristically calmly on my assigned carpet remnant and tumbled the new term over and over in my brain. Nervous.

Our bodies often tell us things about who we are before we know the words for them. Over the next few years, my stomach, heart, and skin let me know I was a "heterosexual," "female" "insomniac" with a tendency toward "depression." That afternoon, I made it my business to confirm what I suspected the term "nervous" meant. It took some doing.

Ordinarily, I'd have asked my mother, but she'd started reacting strangely when I'd ask her innocent questions about words I'd read or overheard.

"Mumsie!" I'd yelled into the kitchen a few months prior (I called her Mumsie—we thought it was fancy and funny. I still do), "The man on the news said a girl got raped. What does 'raped' mean?"

Seconds later, she'd limped into the family room and stooped down to clench my eyes with hers. "Why did you ask that? Those men working on the house next door, have they said something to you? Did they try to talk to you? Did they try to touch you?"

I wrapped my arms around her to soothe her agitation as my own stomach started to flutter. "Nononono. They never talked to me, I promise. Maybe I said hi once to be nice. I'm sorry . . . I'm sorry, Mumsie. Don't worry."

More recently, my TV habit had brought another unexpectedly fraught vocabulary lesson courtesy of the otherwise benign 1960s sitcom *My Three Sons*. Either Fred MacMurray's sage, often-beset widower-with-kids, or the gruff but lovable Uncle Charlie tossed off some crack about needing a psychiatrist.

This time, I'd saved my mother the trip and wandered into the kitchen (she spent a lot of her time in there, but not necessarily for culinary purposes). "Um, what's a psychiatrist?"

I may as well have wandered in juggling a rabid rat, a live chain saw, and a phonics test with a red *F* at the top for all the trouble I was suddenly in.

"Don't you DARE tell anyone Mommy sees a psychiatrist! Why would you do that? Who did you tell? It's a secret, and you had no right and everyone will think I'm crazy and . . ."

My dad (Pup, thus named for similar reasons as Mumsie) slid in to soothe her as I slunk off to my room and muffled her cries with a pillow as best I could.

(By the time I saw the word "condom" on a package at the drugstore a few years later, I'd learned to go to the den and consult the family dictionary. Whew.)

I needed neither Mumsie nor *Merriam Webster* to define "nervous," because I knew it simply meant "me," but I come from a people who appreciate empirical evidence and solid source material.

My dad is a Ph.D. chemist, retired now, but still curious to the core. Before I was born, my mother taught recalcitrant high school students to love reading. My sister, whom I call "Nan," emerged from one billion years of higher learning as Dr. Kinsman, Esq., with a Ph.D. in psychology and a law degree to boot. I'm the academic slacker in the bunch with a master's degree in metalsmithing, but still, I had to log some library time in addition to smashing brass with hammers.

And so, that afternoon I did as I'd been taught by a family prone to settling dinnertime disputes with a trip to the den to grab a reference book. That seems incredibly quaint now in our information-glutted era, but it was a sufficient argument-ender well into the nineties—and pretty damned definitive.

So far as I could stitch together from the dictionary, the *N* volume of the *Encyclopedia Britannica* and some consumer-friendly analog of *Gray's Anatomy,* "nervous" fit my jittery hands like custom-sewn gloves. The searing stomach, the quickened pulse, the full-body fear, knocking knees, and closed-up throat—I finally had a word I could wield when someone asked what was wrong with me. Over the next few decades, I did. A lot.

"Nervous" accounted for my like-clockwork nausea on the nights before the first day of school or a new soccer season. It vindicated my jittery test-day hands and their tendency to pick at my skin until blood streamed down and stained my sleeves and socks.

On the days when my mother was in the hospital for one of her seemingly endless knee, back, and foot surgeries, it explained away the acidic stabs of my stomach. Those were so severe that I'd spend recess hunched in a ball by the Dumpster while my friends played freeze tag on the blacktop until some adult was dispatched to assess my well-being.

"Katie, are you all right?"

"Uh-huh. My mom is in the hospital. I'm just nervous for her, I guess."

"I'm so sorry. You tell her we're all praying for her. Now, why don't you go try to play and forget about it for right now, okay?"

"Okay. Thank you, Sister Mary."

I'd try to seem better for their benefit, throw myself into the chaos and clamor of the games that seemed to delight my friends. I knew it wasn't actually going to work—you know from early on of what material you're built—but I didn't want the guilt of someone else's worry about me to pull me down further into the muck.

If I couldn't hide my upset, I'd do my best to pin it to a solvable problem. It just worked best for everyone that way. Fretting about a test? Okay, you can skip doing the dishes so you can go study. Your mom is sick? I'll say a prayer for her.

But it's a different beast when there's no solution, no clear cause and effect—when there's no triggering incident that makes you stop washing your hair because you're suddenly terrified at the prospect of getting your head wet.

When you show up at school with bruise-brown circles under your eyes because you were terrified Satan would possess your idle mind in your sleep (or that's at least how you'd interpreted that day's Bible study).

When you start brown-bagging lunch because you've become afraid that cafeteria food will make you sick to your stomach.

When you're not nervous because of anything; you're just nervous.

You can't tell anyone, because that's just crazy. And that's a secret.

IRRATIONAL FEAR #1
HAVING NO WAY OUT

I spent my childhood walking slowly, keeping pace with my mother no matter how glacially she moved, as she needed to coddle her arthritic joints to keep them from screaming. This may partially explain why as an adult, and a resident of New York City for nearly two decades, I now slip silverfish quickly down crowded streets, air frozen in my throat when I'm penned in by anyone ambling, less urgent, or simply unable. Walkwalkwalkwalkdammitwalk. My brain sparks with a fury as I dart around them the second I see an opening. When quarters get too close, on the street, on the subway, I pop out my earbuds because I can't spare the focus. I must keep my eyes on the escape routes or I can't breathe.

"Stop walking like a damn Yankee!" a friend chirped at me recently as we walked a Mississippi street. I'm pretty sure I'd walk that way no matter where I'd made my home as an adult, but let's go with the Yankee tag for now. And as it is, I only really feel at ease in my home—my apartment, specifically. The rest of the time I spend feeling tugged toward it.

This is the fight-or-flight part of my anxiety disorder, I guess. I know the *toward*, but the *from* can vary. Usually it's people. Strangers. Bodies stuffed into subway cars until we're molded together shoulder to shoulder, backpack to kidney, face to crotch (seriously), and I'm certain I'm going to miss my stop because they're blocking my way to the door. I'll sit at my desk for an extra twenty minutes, forty, two hours, blood sugar dropping and Douglas pacing the floors waiting for me at home because I'm dreading the crush of rush hour. Escalators can do it, too, especially in cities where walking may not be the primary mode of transport and the standard pace is molasses-like. Standing on one—rather than actually treating it as a moving staircase—makes the blood prickle at my temples until I can explode free at the top or bottom. The thought of a slowly emptying concert lobby after the final encore is making my throat close up right now.

Unless I am fixed in place somewhere comfortable in my home, or sufficiently distracted by a task, a good meal, or scintillating conversation, the bulk of my brain matter is fixated on how the hell I'm going to get out of there. It's not always conscious; in fact, I'd say that by this point, it's an automatic reflex, like a heartbeat or breathing. And somehow it's become just as fundamental to my staying alive—at least the way my twitchy brain has worked it.

Maybe I've spent too much time around rabbits. I've adopted a few scared, traumatized, rehabbed bunnies over the past dozen years. Here, they never had to worry about where their next mouthful of hay was coming from or if my hands were poised to do anything other than stroke their body to a purr, but it was bred into their bones that they should flee. The rabbits and I share that genetic trait. We always know the way out. Follow me to safety. Or actually . . . don't. I need some air.

Mortifyingly enough, a few seconds too long in a zipper-stuck dress, or with a scarf (even my own hair) wound over my mouth, or a coat that's taking too long to unbutton makes me almost feral, afraid that I'll never breathe freely again.

This fear of being pinned in place, deprived of oxygen, or unexpectedly groped from the back (which *has* happened more than once in public and private, so this ain't coming from nowhere) unconsciously informs my physical placement nearly anywhere I go. Movie theater: back row, aisle. Center if the theater is empty-ish (which whenever possible is when I go). Subway: stand 85 percent of the time, near a door when able. Never take a middle seat. Plane: exit row, window, left-hand side if available. (The aisle passengers filing past during boarding make my brain practically short-circuit.) Standing-room-only concert: way up at the front, back against a wall or on a balcony (I will always opt for a balcony if I can). IKEA, Target, and great big grocery stores: only on weekdays. Parades and the Rockefeller Center tree lighting: HAHAHAHAHAHA. ARE YOU KIDDING?!

Parties are a particular conundrum because in theory, I'm attending because I'd love to spend time with the host and/or the other invitees. But "parties"—especially in my line of work—often blur the boundary between the social and the professional. And there's usually booze, which helps or hurts depending on who's consumed it and how much.

I don't know if a flute (or a vat) of Prosecco would have bubbled my troubles away the first time I had a panic attack in public—in front of nonstrangers—that I couldn't hide. It was at Lincoln Center in the press room for the James Beard Awards at the start of my food-writing career. While I was there to file a story on the winners, word quickly spread that the smallish room was the place to be for chefs (and their entourages) to avoid the scrum and raise a glass after their category had been called. I can't pretend I wasn't a little star-struck seeing my food idols up close and personal . . . and then very, very up close. Dammit. I'd stepped away from my laptop (not quite corner, table facing the wall) to stretch and grab a drink on the other side of the room, and in the meantime, the path back to my home base had filled up with swaying, sweating, celebrating bodies. I breathed. I grounded my feet. I made small talk with an acquaintance. Then it happened.

A woman made eye contact, nailed a smile onto her face, and strode over. "You. You never answer my e-mails, but here you are. Let's chat." She was a publicist, it turned out. One I'd never met or answered because she'd yet to pitch me anything I could actually use. But there she was, in the cocktail-dress-bedecked flesh, making the most of the moment. She closed in, standing inches from me, blocking me in against the wall, talkingtalkingtalking, and getting taller by the second. Or so it seemed. My acquaintance (now a friend) tells me that I pressed my back up against the wall and slid down centimeter by centimeter, smiling and nodding the whole way, until the woman was just standing over me, delivering her spiel as I crouched on the floor in my party dress. All I recall is my field of vision narrowing to a gray cone and the heat of the room barreling into my face and chest until it shoved me onto the carpet. Eventually, this friend wedged his way between us, distracted her, and created a shield for me with his tuxedoed body until I could regain my composure for the moment—at least on the outside. My pulse raced for the rest of the night and I just felt spent and mortified to have lost it so visibly in front of my professional peers. (He swears no one noticed. He's a very kind man.)

Since then, I scope out any crowded space, constantly running mental calculations on every other person's place in space and where they might move next.

Can I afford to slip back to refill my glass, or will bodies trap me in my friend's galley kitchen for the rest of the party?

I really want to go into that tiny bakery, but there's a child on a scooter doing laps inside while his mother sips her latte, obliviously. Do I dare risk my toes and/or sanity for the sake of some gingerbread? (It's really good gingerbread.)

If I move farther toward the center of this train car, will that family with the shopping bags and guy with the bike (seriously, guy—did you have to haul that on during rush hour?) pen me in so I'll miss my stop?

That was my boarding zone they called, but all these people are crowded around the door and theirs hasn't yet been called. If I thread through and board when I'm supposed to, will they all be glaring at the jerk in 13A for the rest of the flight, tweeting their hopes for my swift, non-plane-crash-related demise?

I know the look on the face of the semistranger walking toward me at this work event—they're going to ask me a million unintentionally invasive questions usually about my mental health state (because I've been public about it, and they really want to know for themselves, and I understand that and want to help, and I wrote those articles, but . . .) and trap me in this corner away from the snack table where I was headed because my blood sugar is dipping by the minute. How do I gracefully bolt before they reach me? Or at least get a few hors d'oeuvres into my gaping maw before I have to respond? (Actually, the move I've perfected lately is saying, "Hey, I was on my way to the food. Come with me?" So I'm vaguely less cranky, less trapped, and better fed.)

I tried once to shock myself out of this fear, take it to such an extreme that anything after would seem like a cakewalk in contrast. I couched it as a piece of performance art at a fetish party (we'll get to that): having my boyfriend strip me down to my underwear in front of a crowd, then bind my whole body, mummy-style, in plastic wrap while I lay on a bench in a basement. There was a slit for my nose and mouth. I may be an emotional masochist, but I shy away from actual physical harm. Exposed in public and completely confined at the same time—this was pretty much my worst nightmares made flesh. I fell asleep, likely due to the lack of circulation. Or perhaps it was the emotional overload of succumbing to the idea that there was absolutely nothing I could do to save myself—and that every single bit of the horror was self-inflicted.

I suppose living in New York is self-inflicted; taking the train, walking the body-packed streets, all scrambling for the same supplies and confining ourselves to stacked-up quarters that are dwarfed in size by suburban toddlers' bedrooms. But I hear that people in other cities have parties and escalators, too. And crowded stores and airports and well-meaning people in pain who just need to recharge themselves from someone else's battery for a moment with a conversation.

I can't outrun any of it, I guess.

Come and get me.

CHAPTER TWO

All in the Family

In sixth grade, my parents, teachers, and doctors all decided I was sick with mono. There was no real test for this ailment (at least at the time), and a couple of kids at a neighboring school had come down with what we all called the kissing disease, which so far as I understood was supposed to make you feel tired, and tender about the spleen. I'd no idea where my spleen was (and surely hadn't been doing any kissing), but was grateful for any respite from the hell that was my school day.

Oddly enough, I'd finally made an alliance with Lana, a long-time nemesis, when I point-blank asked why she hated me so much. She countered with the same question. It turns out we each just wanted what the other had—popularity (her) and academic accolades (me)—and once it had been said aloud, we curled our pinkie fingers together and swore ourselves friends. Such are the strange, changeable politics of eleven-year-old girls.

But all the warm will of a new friend couldn't save me from Mrs. S, who could not bear the thought of a child rising above their station, thinking well of themselves, or bothering with such silliness as friendships or alliances.

In my mind, she cast a shadow the size of a china closet, heaving her arthritic bulk to loom over the desk of students she felt needed special correction. Other times, she barked and boomed across the room, letting her displeasure echo against the wall of stunned silence.

I was stupid enough to cross her once, challenging her on a fact I knew she'd gotten wrong. I'd just watched some World War I documentary with my dad and was armed with the information. The geek in me just couldn't let it stand. I shot. She fired back. Hers landed.

Since then, I've learned an awful lot of lessons about picking the hills upon which I'm willing to die. I chose poorly that day and, in the following months, was treated to a daily dose of displeasure from my teacher. Mrs. S had at least one very commendable quality: she was patient and kind with students who had a tough time learning. Even through my veil of terror, I couldn't help but admire the pains to which she went to make sure that every kid could keep up (even if I suspected that had to do with the fact that one of them was her grandson).

But it also meant she had to knock the tall poppies down. No matter how invisible I tried to make myself, in how small a ball I tried to curl, she'd find a fresh way every day to shame me—nitpicking my homework, critiquing my appearance, even calling my character into question. Walking into that classroom scraped a little more off my soul each day, and eventually, it breached the surface.

I woke up one morning and simply couldn't move. I was pinned to my bed, unable to breathe. My parents were, of course, worried. They'd seen me felled before, by colds, flu, chicken pox, and other miserable but curable things, and they could sense that something was different. Even now, I hate so much that I put them through that experience—making them share the kitchen table with the sad ghost of the daughter they loved.

And I was sucking the air out of the sickroom Mumsie usually occupied. That's how we lived together in our red-brick suburban house, with her pain pulling up a chair and reclining. We all lived in service or dread of it, because there was no way we could cure it.

I used to make an unfunny joke, because I was young and callow and that's all I knew how to do: if she was a horse, we'd have shot her to put her out of her misery. That is a god-awful thing to say about your own mother, but to hear her cries then, it felt like a kindness. She hurt all the time, from rheumatoid arthritis, fibromyalgia, nerve damage, slipped disks, tongue fissures, and inner-ear issues, off the top of my head. What we didn't know at the time was what was going on inside her head, namely a storm of countless ministrokes mottling her brain and racking her temper from side to side until we all staggered with her, clinging to what we could find for balance.

I don't remember what set her off one Sunday afternoon, just how it scattered us. Nan grabbed her jacket and stomped off to safer ground at her friend's house up the street, disgusted with us all. Pup placed himself right in the eye of it, spiriting Mumsie off to the den, shutting the door and letting her howl at him, "I hurt! I hurt! I hurt!" He'd given me the nod to retreat and I was grateful, but I still felt guilty, shaking my brain for anything I could have done to provoke her pain. Had I been too loud on the stairs last night and disturbed her sleep, said something unpleasant, not jumped up quickly enough to do the dishes? I lay on my bed and clutched a pillow around my head to muffle her increasingly incoherent screams until they subsided. She went to bed early that night and stayed there for a while. We crept through the house, not daring to ripple the air. I still dread Sundays.

But when it was my turn, I went much more quietly. My parents took the mono diagnosis to share with the general public, and at home, my mother set it aside. She was as much in love with words as I was, and no stranger to the symbiosis of body and psyche. After about a week of my lumping around the house, she drew up a chair to the couch where I'd cocooned myself in an afghan and a straight sightline to the TV. Her voice was gentle and measured, as if she were reading a script she'd rehearsed in her head so she wouldn't flub it.

"You know Mrs. S hurts, don't you? She has arthritis, like I do, and she's in pain all the time like me. She might say things because she hurts. She can't help it, so you might just have to be stronger than her sometimes."

I felt myself beginning to evaporate. All my life, I'd seen how much my mother ached—from her knees and her back and from somewhere within, and I loathed that I couldn't lighten that weight for her. I didn't always understand her strange outbursts, but she was my mother and I loved her fiercely, so I'd weather them. But to have to find sympathy for Mrs. S?! That seemed too far to reach.

It wasn't the end of her speech. She reached for my hand to tether me to earth and make sure I heard it, massaging the words in with her worn, bent fingers.

"Don't go away from me. I love you too much. Tell me how to bring you back."

And together that afternoon, we found a word for the thing that had also been consuming me from the inside for as long as I could remember. The word is "gricky."

It won't mean much to anyone else, but it's a portmanteau of "gray" and "icky" and it's what brought me back from the edge then and a thousand times since. Once something has a name, it can be challenged to battle, and if not slain, then at least tamed.

Gricky is a double-headed beast that carries toxic gloom in one set of fangs and electric zaps of panic in the other. When it pounces on top of me—often from nowhere, the stealthy bastard—it fights filthy, sitting on my chest until there's no air left. When it's laid me low, aching from the heart outward, too lead-limbed to move or even blot tears, I still don't rest. Oh hell no. When I'm helplessly pinned in place is when the worry shocks my body hardest.

"You think you're going to sleep now, just because you're in bed in the middle of the afternoon? Ha! Here's the memory of the stupid thing you said at a party, the low grade, the faux pas, the snub, the public tumble. Obsess on that until you finally collapse in exhaustion—then wake in horror remembering all the things you failed to achieve that day. Why are you sucking up all the care and air that someone more worthy could be using? Why do you bother to BE?"

And now I wonder if Mumsie was helping me craft a language of pain because she suspected what was in store for me. I'd found her once, when I was very young and Nan and Pup were out of town overnight for her swim meet, sobbing quietly at the kitchen table. It frightened me to see my mother like that, when I hadn't heard her fall or cut herself, and the telephone hadn't rung with any bad news. I backed away into the family room and tried to stuff my head full of cartoons instead, but when I got to the dinner table, she let me know my cowardice hadn't escaped her notice. "That's not okay. If you see me crying, if you see anyone crying, you ask them what's wrong. That's the right thing to do."

What's wrong was that she was sad. Just because.

I flung myself at her knees and begged for her forgiveness. It occurred to me just a little bit that it was a lot for an adult to expect their grade-schooler to tend to their invisible pain. But maybe since

Pup—the only person who probably knew what her particular "gricky" was—was away, I was the next best thing.

Later on, that language and lesson went through my head a lot in a desperate attempt to self-soothe while watching my mother crumble. So far as I could tell (and as she often told me), I was at the core of her worry, and my impending departure for college was what was causing it to escalate. She didn't mean it, but she got mean. She blamed it on the pain, she blamed it on me. I did, too. I didn't know any better.

On a day Pup and I were supposed to fly to Baltimore to visit the college I would eventually attend, she had a panic attack so bad that we had to reschedule the trip. When I did eventually leave, she spent the morning with her church singing group rehearsing in our kitchen, lofting praises unto the heavens while I stuffed my record collection and thrift-shop dresses into the car. She waved good-bye to me from the sidewalk.

And a few weeks later, my new roommate handed me the phone. "Don't worry," Pup said, "she's alive, but . . ."

He brought her home a few weeks later, with a mighty pharmaceutical cocktail to keep the urges and worry away, as well as a diagnosis that for the first time hung heavily on the word "anxiety."

And I ran like hell from it—from her—for a long, long time.

When someone attempts not to be your mother anymore, the natural response would be trying to prove how much you are not like them, no matter how much you love them. For me, that's not an option, and I've stopped trying to fight it. It's simply not winnable.

We look so much alike, it's undeniable that we are mother and daughter, even though my face is animated to the point of cartoonishness, and hers has slipped into a stony mask from lack of dopamine. My knuckles have begun to gnarl just slightly, in an achingly familiar way, and when my mouth twists up to laugh, it's an echo of her from what feels like a lifetime ago.

Mumsie can't laugh much anymore. Or speak much, or read much or write or teach or any of the other things that gave her pleasure and carved her place in the world. Parkinson's disease, Lewy body dementia, and decades of small strokes have ravaged her memory centers and shrunk her world to the range of her wheelchair and the size of her nursing-home bed. Honestly, I'm not always sure she knows who I am.

But I do.

I'm Kat. I'm my Mumsie's daughter. We have anxiety.

But it doesn't have me.

CHAPTER THREE

School Days

When we were in the eighth grade, Elle stood outside my kitchen at dinnertime and listened through the screen door for anything she could use as a weapon against me. She was short, bony, fair-haired, and eternally tan, and our friends had long ago nicknamed me "Casper" in contrast. We'd started out as foes in kindergarten when we both had a crush on the same boy and ever after cycled through phases of sworn enmity and pinkie-locking besties. Over the years, she'd developed a particular knack for finding the thinnest parts of my skin, scraping them sore, then administering a butterfly kiss to make it all better. It's an odd, toxic skill that some girls have, find-ing another girl's vulnerabilities and helping her "correct" them in the name of friendship. And we were friends by then—she'd made sure of it, after years of silent and not so silent torment. My connec-tion to her best friend, Lana, made it impossible for Elle to publicly hate me any longer, and as Lana would be starting at a different high school than us in the fall, Elle declared me the third leg of the trio. Her "other" best friend, even. With this declaration, it became harder for me to get mad at her—and easier for her to get to me.

From the kitchen-door surveillance, she picked up private family nicknames and jokes to embarrass me with in front of a crowd. She had come over to "congratulate" me for some academic honor, then calmly took a garden hose, aimed it through the open windows of our dining room, and soaked everything inside. I screamed, sick to my stomach that my parents would be angry with me. When I went outside, she told me she was no longer my friend. I chased her down the street, begging for forgiveness.

Our religion teacher assigned an exercise, handing out slips of paper, each inscribed with the quality of a good Christian person: generosity, kindness, patience, etc. Then we were told to put our slip of paper on the desk of the person who most possessed that quality. All but a couple ended up on my desk. Elle got none.

She invited me to her house for a sleepover that weekend and walked around me in a circle hissing all my secret faults, and smacking and flicking my arms, back, and neck so they'd sink into my balled-up body and leave a mark. She told me to thank her. I did.

She knew I worried—I'd never made a secret of it and couldn't hide it if I tried—but she did her best to make sure I had plenty to worry about. Then maybe my focus would slip and my performance would stumble so her parents would stop bothering her about why she didn't have my good grades or my spot on the cheerleading squad at our new high school. This was a chance for both of us to reinvent ourselves outside the small circle of kids we'd known since kindergarten. New friends wouldn't have to know that I'd been cheerleading since fifth grade, gotten good at it, even, because I was too clumsy to make the basketball team. Maybe it would blind them to my fundamental dorkiness, and they'd never have to know that my short hair—which my mother insisted on—used to occasionally make me be mistaken for a boy. Maybe I could meet people who could see something lovable or worthy in me that wasn't just based on my grades.

Elle was convinced she could finally be on top. She hated her own nose, so she'd grasp mine and yank while telling me how hideous my face was, and then offer a hairstyling tip as a bit of kindness. She made up a dance, stitched together from all my nervous tics of shaking hands and hair twisting, and tried to teach it to the other kids (who, to their credit, told her it was pretty mean) so she could show me what I needed to fix. She'd pull me outside at lunchtime or down into her basement after school to tell me how worthless and awkward and unlikable I was, what freaks she found my family to be, and how everyone else did, too, but she was my best friend and the only one who cared enough to tell me and get me ready for how cruel the rest of the world was going to be to me. She taught me one thing: to flinch and brace, even if there was no fist coming my way.

In 1986, when I was thirteen years old, I traveled to Washington, D.C., to compete in the National Spelling Bee. I had already been dealing with the physical effects of anxiety since I was too young to really know what was going on, but the pressure of this situation was like nothing I had ever experienced. To this day, I cannot watch the Bee on TV without my throat closing up, and my nerves were in such a frazzled state at the time, my dad, having done some light reading on Maharishi Mahesh Yogi, made Transcendental Meditation a part of our regular practice sessions. (Note: it was mostly lost on me, but I take comfort in the occasional "ohm.") This is an excerpt from the diary I kept during the days I spent there. Clearly Elle's lessons had sunk in. God forbid I give myself a pat on the back for having made it all that way. The only positive outcomes: win (and heaven help me if I did that), or be a massive disappointment to everyone who had put their faith in me.

Diary Entry: May 28, 1986

Suffice it to say I almost lost my awful Egg McMuffin in the first round. I had no idea that it would take this kind of toll on my body. We were in our seats at eight fifteen, they didn't stop talking until a nerve-racking nine. It was then only the practice round and people were already out for blood. I mean we knew our words and they would already ask for everything. One boy says, "Please define" like a robot, another says, *"C"*—five-minute pause—*"A"*—five minutes—"can I start over? *C* . . ."

I made it through without fainting, but afterward, during the break, I looked for something long and sharp with which to stab myself. Preferably a [*sic*] hari-kari knife. The round took over an hour. Karla invited me to go to her room that night. The hugs from Mom and Linda Parker (the reporter who was traveling with us to cover the event for the *Kentucky Post,* which was sponsoring my trip) do wonders. I got up there for the first round. The wait was interminable. The relief was unbelievable when the first girl got out. She was in agony, at the mercy of the long, grabbing microphones. The relief didn't last long. I was in agony now, waiting for my turn. I was at the mercy of the octopus of grabbing microphones and glaring lights.

A disembodied voice said "ethos" and it was like what I imagine Judgment Day will be like. I asked for a definition and went into a daze. Somehow, I spelled it right and went back and fogged out in my seat. We went to Hardee's. I had a really awful lunch. I was too keyed up to eat.

And so went the report filed by the aforementioned Ms. Parker to the *Post* later that afternoon:

ARACHIN. SACCHARIMETER. FEIJO. AND PHYLLOPHOROUS.

Those words, and others like them, claimed 59 spellers in the Scripps Howard National Spelling Bee Wednesday. Katie Kinsman, *Kentucky Post* champion, was among them.

But she turned in a championship performance.

"I've never seen her this nervous," her mother, Dottie Kinsman of Fort Thomas, said Wednesday morning, before the 59th annual bee began. Her coach and father, Donald, was "so nervous he couldn't watch," said Katie. "He can never watch me in competitions."

Under hot lights and through more than two hours of ceremonies and a practice round, the 13-year-old eighth grader from St. Thomas School sat on stage with 173 other spellers sponsored by newspapers across the country.

Finally, as speller no. 100, she got to spell her first official word: "ethos."

No problem. Still, "I'm nervous the whole time," she said after the first round Wednesday. She managed those nerves through a lunch break and another hour of sitting and listening, while spellers in front of her missed such words as "verricule" and "oceandromous."

It was her turn.

"Fuh-LOFF-er-us," said pronouncer Dr. Alex Cameron of the University of Dayton, Ohio. Katie asked for the definition, and was told it was an adjective meaning "leaf bearing." She took a deep breath and spelled "filoferous." The judges hit an old-fashioned desk bell, and Katie was escorted offstage to the "crying room."

The initial disappointment was bitter, but Katie quickly demonstrated the maturity and sunny grace that have been her hallmarks during her Post-sponsored week in Washington.

"This is a bummer," she said, brushing a few tears from her face. "I really wanted to make it to the fourth round." She quickly squared her shoulders. "Okay. I guess I'm okay." With her mother's arm around her, Katie said, "Well, now I guess I don't have to be nervous anymore . . . but I was kind of hoping I'd get one I knew . . . but I guess I should be proud I made it here . . . Okay now. I'm fine," she said, jumping up and approaching the other spellers in the room.

"I know she's dreading facing the gang at home," her mother said. "But she'll recover quickly. I'm just thrilled she was able to come here and have this experience. It broadens her and us."

Within moments, Katie was back in the crowded hall, consoling other spellers who shared her fate and cheering on friends who still remained in competition . . .

Diary Entry: May 29, 1986

These kids are in sheer hell! You cry with them when they get out. You share their happiness when they triumph. Me especially. I was one of them yesterday. These words make no sense. The only time they are used is here. Why do we do this to ourselves?

If I'd let myself see me through the reporter's eyes, I wonder if I could have spared myself the next few years of worrying that I was failing everyone, all the time, simply by existing. I wasn't up there to win. I stood under those unforgiving klieg lights with my terrible perm, brace-faced grimace, and acid stomach for the express purpose of proving my worth, and I couldn't. And now I had to go back and face everyone I'd let down.

Linda saw something else—the worth of a kid who could step past her own disappointment and cheer on someone who still needed it. But that's not cool or cute when you're thirteen. It doesn't make your crush check "like" on a passed note, seat you at the popular table, or make your fake Jordache skirt hug your nonexistent curves just so. It makes you a loser—a word that wouldn't have applied to you if you'd just stuck to the sidelines and never had the audacity to compete in the first place.

One guess as to who made sure several months later that everyone in the freshman class at our new high school knew that "weirdo" should be attached to my name. Not that they actually used it—at least not to my face. But Elle started up a targeted campaign to make sure I believed they did. Unsigned notes left in my locker spelled out how ugly and strange I was. (I caught her once and she claimed someone told her to put it in there.) Hissed threats made me dread the sound of the telephone, back when *69 and caller ID were yet a twinkle in Ma Bell's eye. And ugh, lunch inevitably came served with a steaming side of verbal abuse, dished out of earshot of nearby authority figures. I couldn't possibly have choked down the slab of industrial pizza on the menu that day because I'd already swallowed Elle's message whole: Everyone thinks you're awkward, unattractive, and strange. I'm telling you this because I'm the only one who cares about you enough to be honest.

I let all of this happen because somehow I was sure Elle was right. She gave audible voice and physical force to the thing inside me that told me that I was less than. I was too tired to fight any longer. When you're mentally ill, you learn quickly how to compartmentalize because God forbid anyone figure out that you're crazy. It's too shameful and you don't want to burden anyone else (say, your sick mother) with it. You paste on a smile. You shake your pom-poms. You leap and twirl and cheer until you fall from the sky.

I eventually stopped going to school in ninth grade ("mono" again), inflicting my wretchedness only on the people in my family, and using up the air and sunlight that should by all rights be used by someone more worthy of them than me.

Words, for once, failed me. One day, laid flat at the bottom of a flight of stairs I was too tired to climb, I spared three of the very few I had left: "I need help."

In exchange, I got a new one: "depression."

It was given to me by my brand-new psychiatrist, Dr. Merwin, along with a bottle of rhino-sized pills, and permission to blame my body instead of my being. I flushed the pills (mid-1980s tricyclics that left me dry-mouthed, constipated, and dizzy), but grasped on to the label, which I found oddly freeing, and naively, exotic.

"Depression" wasn't, in my mind, the stuff of boring, ordinary suburban teens; it was the mantle of the tortured writers I'd always idolized. And if I had to suffer the lows, I might as well reap the spoils—the chief of them being not having to give a flying crap about what the Elles of the world thought anymore.

God, it was bliss not caring, for the first time in my life feeling unapologetic about who I was, how I looked, and what I loved to do. I quit the cheerleading squad, dressed how I wanted, and drank coffee in diners all night with new friends who appreciated my Monty Python and Douglas Adams jokes.

As high school went on, I did my best to pay it forward, too—

listening between the lines as best I could to schoolmates who seemed as if they were trying to stretch a lip-glossed smile over some serious wounds, and letting them know they weren't alone. Turns out that even the pretty people see shrinks and take pills. A freak like me just had less to lose by talking openly about it.

I even had it in me to forgive Elle, who materialized at my feet one day during our high school's mandatory spiritual retreat a week or two before graduation. As we sat in yawning contemplation in the chapel, Father Somethingorother yea and verily decreed that we should seek the forgiveness of anyone who we had harmed so that we could stride into our futures pure of heart and light of soul.

I rolled my eyes and scribbled in my journal until I suddenly heard a small, snuffling sound in the aisle next to my pew. It was Elle, crouched down on her knees, sobbing quietly and whispering, "I'm so sorry . . . I'm so sorry . . ." over and over again.

I'd dreamed of this moment a million times what seemed like a lifetime ago, plotted my icy comebacks, imagined delivering the same physical humiliations she'd inflicted on me. But all I felt in that moment was . . . human. She was a scared, small, awkward girl and to repay the pain at this point would come at a cost to the person I was becoming.

I gave her the only thing I could afford: "It's okay. Don't worry. I'm okay."

IRRATIONAL FEAR #2
DANCING

In four hours, 661 miles from where I'm sitting, my twenty-five-year high school reunion will begin. I could toss a dress, shoes, and lipstick in a bag (trusting drugstores there to provide the rest), grab a cab, spend just shy of a thousand bucks, and get there just as the sun sets over the banks of the Ohio River at the camp where the celebration is being held. (BYO bottle, snack, and chair, and we'll pass a hat for the band.) In theory, I could do all of these things. But I won't. Not this year or the fifteen that have passed since I last attended one of these events. I don't loathe or fear anyone. Not actively. Not anymore. That faded with the rise of Facebook when I could see—really see—my former tormentors for what they really were: people. Not Dementors or a special army of black-ops soldiers specifically trained to smash-killdestroy my self-esteem. They are, like me, just ex-dumbshit and terrified teens who were just trying to weather the world and personal circumstances as best they could. Plenty of them have even turned out to be quite knowing, as adults.

That doesn't mean I want to dance in front of them.

Yeah, that platitude about "Dance like no one is watching!" means bubkes unless Jack Daniel's and Jim Beam are flanking me in the reception kick line. The path from my chair to the thick of the dance floor has not worn smooth with the passage of time, and of all of life's supposedly simple pleasures that anxiety robs me of, I'm perhaps most pissed off about this one.

I wasn't always this way, a chorophobic (the technical term for someone who fears dancing). I danced with abandon as a kid, encouraged in no small part by Pup, who though he staunchly refused to boogie down in public would in private perform a marvelously silly, slack-faced, paws-up, shuffling "doggie dance" that still makes me light up every time it comes to mind.

God, back then I'd sing in public, too, and tell jokes over the intercom at the YMCA and play the piano (I specialized in very heartfelt renditions of TV theme songs) for anyone, with the slightest bit of provocation. I was terrified of plenty of things, but never ashamed to put these "talents" on display, until suddenly I was. Maybe it's inevitable once a girl hits an especially self-conscious age, but it was actually done to me, thieved from me deliberately, and I am mortified that I haven't high-kicked in to take it back.

"Everyone is making fun of you." That's all it took at age thirteen to still my dancing feet and fling me to the walls to cling on for safety. It was the middle of an eighth-grade dance when Elle (who else?) pulled me aside to demonstrate the acceptable way to groove along to a song from the *Purple Rain* sound track—not the wild-limbed, low-gravity moves I thought the music had told me to bust, but rather an in-place, side-to-side shuffle with sheepish snaps and claps to accentuate any enthusiasm. Exactly who had found my movements so aesthetically objectionable, she declined to say, but the notion of anyone or, yikes, EVERYONE—

1. Actually noticing me.
2. Passing judgment on how I moved my body in times of joy.

—was upsetting, to say the least. I slumped my shoulders, hung my head.

I didn't think to question her or simply trust that my arms, legs, pelvis, and chest wanted to move that way. The next years as a high school cheerleader and school-musical chorus-line dancer, I clutched on to the choreography like a kickboard. If I executed the preordained steps perfectly, no one could see anything of the real me through the twirls and bounds. If someone—usually a coach or someone's mom—complimented me, I'd tell them thank you, and just assume they were in on the joke, too.

But once you're past the age of high school athletics, there aren't all that many opportunities for synchronized movement, and I just . . . stilled. I assumed that everyone knew why. Who would want to see *her* move to the groove? She offends. Pluck her out.

At my wedding, I spared both Pup and myself the indignity—no father-daughter dance—telling myself that it would be cruel to leave Mumsie adrift for those moments. It was touch and go that she'd actually make it to the event at all, so why add extra worry for either of them? Or for my new husband; Douglas used to dance professionally (occasionally on top of a box or in a cage on a popular nineties cable show . . .), and I did not wish for him to spend our wedding day stewing in the horror that he was shackled to a mortifying dancer for all of eternity. So, there was also no formal first dance at the affair either, just me attributing my lack of movement to the cinch of my corset and the bulk of sixty-four yards of red tulle. (I did spin a few times because, come on: sixty-four yards of red tulle with black flames licking up from the bottom!)

Douglas knows why now, and we dance at home, constantly and goofily. It's one of my favorite parts of our marriage. But with rare exceptions, like the confluence of drawn curtains, the company of exceptionally close friends, and stunning quantities of Prosecco, it remains a very private indulgence. The notion of moving my body uninhibited in the presence of someone who might mock it makes me sick to my stomach. (In my personal inferno, the innermost ring is a dance circle into whose center I am flung—but at least I wouldn't be alone. Johnny Depp confessed on *The Ellen DeGeneres Show* that his phobia is so severe that he'd "rather swallow a bag of hair" than dance in public out of character and unchoreographed.)

Of all my fears, this is probably the one that practically impacts my life the least (well, save for the whole wedding work-around), but upsets me proportionately more. It's a direct denial of happiness for the sake of . . . I'm no longer sure. A chorus of ghosts, I guess. But no more. I've decided that this one, I'm going to get up, get down, and fight.

I lost a friend recently, suddenly and shockingly. He lived life boisterously, without apology, driving people mad, and to places of unexpected delight. There is a video of the night before he died—a 4 A.M. karaoke belt-out of "Islands in the Stream" in the midst of friends, rough and joyous. The next evening, word of his passing traveled through the press room of the awards show we had all gathered to attend. No one wanted to believe it, least of all those who had seen him living so aggressively just sixteen hours before. And none of us knew what to do, wafting around in tuxedoes and cocktail dresses, offering cheers to the victors, wondering when it would be acceptable to crumble.

Then a friend texted—come to this restaurant, just a few of us hanging out. I headed over, not ready to be alone yet. They'd prepped for a victory, but found themselves weathering a loss, and by the time I arrived, slouching through the early-May Chicago mist, the wine was done and I didn't want any anyway. I grabbed a bottle of San Pellegrino and swung it over my head as we all started to dance, because honestly, we couldn't think of what else to do—and I'm pretty damned sure he'd have done the same thing.

No one laughed at me. They simply joined in.

I may not make it to my reunion tonight (and seriously, for a thousand-dollar trip I'd at least like some passed hors d'oeuvres and a Solo cup fulla trash-can punch), but for my thirty-year, I just might find my dancing feet squelching in the mud alongside the mighty Ohio, letting the music carry me away. And I hope I won't give a crap who's watching.

CHAPTER FOUR

The Number of the Beast

300.02 is the number of my beast. It's *The Diagnostic and Statistical Manual of Mental Disorders* (*DSM-5*) classification code for generalized anxiety disorder (GAD), and it's clawed its way into the top slot as the most frequently diagnosed mental illness in the United States of America (USA). According to the American Psychiatric Association (APA), more than twenty-five million Americans are affected by anxiety disorders.

By the calculations of the Anxiety and Depression Association of America (ADAA), there are some forty million Americans eighteen and older—that's 18 percent of the adult population—who have been clinically anointed with anxiety-related mental health conditions. 22.8 percent of these cases (4.1 percent of the U.S.'s adult population) are considered "severe." By the National Institute of Mental Health's (NIMH) count (and everyone else's), generally anxious women outnumber generally anxious men roughly two to one. Huzzah for the ladies, cosmopolitans and chocolate all around.

The scope of the diagnosis doesn't really shock me, and in fact, I'm surprised the number's not a good deal higher. While we live in advanced and chatty times, by all accounts—instant communication with loved (and loathed) ones at the swipe of a finger, wrist-borne devices that clue us in to our sleep efficiency and step count, the ability to know what any given celebrity is drinking at the club or on their hotel balcony within minutes of their first sip—mo' data doesn't necessarily mean mo' serenity. In fact, it's probably the exact opposite.

But let's start with a clinical definition of anxiety. Per the APA, the auteurs of the *DSM-5*, generalized anxiety disorder entails ongoing, severe tension that interferes with daily functioning. Related anxious conditions include panic disorder and agoraphobia (both of which I also suffer from to some degree), social anxiety disorder or social phobia, obsessive-compulsive disorder (OCD), post-traumatic stress disorder (PTSD), and specific phobias like flying (aviophobia), spiders (arachnophobia), and pinaciphobia (lists), all with a duration of at least six months. There is as yet no clinical term for "fear of acronyms," but you have my apologies if you suddenly feel like you're coming down with a mild case of it.

So clearly, this isn't just your garden-variety case of nerves.

"What are you nervous about?"

"I am nervous about paying my bills / the results of this pregnancy test / my kid driving alone after dark for the first time."

"Those are all sane and healthy things to be nervous about. Carry on, nervous person!"

Fear is good. Fear is logical. Fear is what keeps us from snapping selfies with grizzly bears, turning cartwheels near cliff edges, walking down unlit alleyways, and waiting until the morning-of to study for the SAT. Some quantify fear as a gift that keeps us from exposing ourselves to potential violence, but the kind of worry we're talking about is magnified to such a degree that it becomes an act of violence upon one's own soul.

And body, too. For purposes of an anxiety or phobia diagnosis, a person must have been suffering from the condition for at least six months and the previous edition of the *DSM* (now stricken from the *DSM-5*) required that sufferers "must recognize that their fear and anxiety are excessive or unreasonable." But for a person who's ever endured a panic attack or the debilitating effects of multiple sleepless nights on their workday, six weeks, six days, six hours, or even six minutes can seem like a small trip to hell. Common physical symptoms include stomach upset (the stomach's hundred-million-neuron enteric nervous system reacts independently from the brain, and 90 percent of the fibers in the nerve that connects the two carry information upward from the gut, as opposed to in the other direction) and "butterflies" (caused by a restriction in blood flow because the pituitary and adrenal glands are too busy upping your heart rate and blood pressure), a pounding heart, increased startle reflexes, and muscle tension—none of which are especially conducive to getting the sort of rest required to deal with anxiety in a rational manner. This can have profound effects on work or school performance, interpersonal relationships, and the normal business of everyday life. And failures (real or imagined) on that front can often lead to more worry—and far too often, self-medication with booze or illicit substances. Most people get a nervous tummy or a bout of insomnia from time to time, but for an awful lot of us anxious folks, it's just our baseline state of being.

If that isn't festive enough, there are also panic attacks: a delightful pas de deux of physical and psychological symptoms so intense that the sufferer becomes overwhelmed, and may feel as if they are dying or going crazy. According to the APA, a panic attack may include: pounding heart or chest pain, sweating, trembling, shaking, shortness of breath, sensation of choking, nausea or abdominal pain, dizziness or light-headedness, feeling unreal or disconnected, fear of losing control, "going crazy" (not in the fun Prince way) or dying, numbness, chills, or hot flashes. It's not unheard of for a first-time panic-attack-haver to rush to the nearest emergency room for fear that they are suffering a heart attack or some other life-threatening illness, only to be handed some Ativan and a number for a mental health professional.

Some people may experience only one in their lifetime (and that's PLENTY), but weather a bunch of them (like I do) and you've got a panic disorder. They may be triggered by specific things (driving, crowds, clowns, crowds of driving clowns) or just pop out of thin air, leaving some sufferers to have panic attacks because they fear having, well, a panic attack. The anticipatory anxiety becomes a vicious cycle that can usher in some protective behaviors that, left unchecked, can become phobias themselves. They may stop seeing family or friends because the fear of a panic attack while flying or driving is too intense, shopping in certain stores because it would entail an escalator or elevator trip, eating in restaurants where they are convinced they were given food poisoning—and then in any restaurants at all. Roughly one third of people who suffer from panic disorder end up dealing with some degree of agoraphobia, leaving them unable to operate outside a safety zone that may be as large as a surrounding neighborhood, or as small as a single room in their home, where, unfortunately, they may still suffer from panic attacks—now compounded by an inability to leave and seek treatment. (Not all agoraphobics suffer from panic disorder and the two conditions were unlinked in the *DSM-5*.)

And, while general or specific anxiety can appear without warning or as a result of a traumatic experience (firsthand or witnessed domestic violence, pain, assault, natural or man-made disaster, warfare, or other harmful events) at any point in a person's life, clinical evidence shows that some anxiety disorders can begin to manifest in children as young as four—especially conditions like selective mutism (refusing to speak in a situation where it is expected), separation anxiety, and social phobia. The average age of onset for anxiety disorders is eleven. Sure, some of this can be chalked up to standard-issue kid shyness, but for others, it's just the first step on a possibly lifelong journey with a nervous monkey strapped to her or his back.

Here's the good news: Mom, Dad—it's not technically your fault if your kid is jittery almost straight from the womb. There is as yet no definitive evidence that there is a genetic predisposition to anxiety disorders like there is for some conditions including schizophrenia and bipolar disorder. BUT, there is an overwhelming likelihood that environmental factors, especially a parent or two suffering from depression, play a substantial role in the way their offspring learn to process fear. No pressure there.

And there are new factors at play in our highly wired era. In February 2014, Dr. Panpimol Wipulakorn, the deputy director-general of Thailand's department of mental health, warned the country's teenagers that posting selfies on social media sites in the hope of gaining attention and approval was effectively putting them at risk for mental health problems in the future. A study conducted by the psychology department at Michigan State University in 2012 monitored three hundred undergraduates' social media use and found strong evidence that the use of these networks has a direct effect on users' levels of anxiety—both from the added stress of multitasking and from the fear that their lives may suffer in comparison to the ones they see their peers representing online. (It is worth noting that several mental health professionals associated with the study also suggested that anxious people may be more prone to overusing social media in the first place, depending on it as a substitute for in-person interactions.) But it's not just those crazy kids getting their knickers in a twist on the interwebs. A 2013 *Today* show survey of seven thousand mothers revealed that 42 percent of them suffered from what they called "Pinterest stress," or the worry that they weren't as creative or crafty as the other moms who were whipping up handmade party favors and Martha-worthy cupcakes to display on the photo networking site. A quarter of the respondents indicated that the self-imposed pressure to be perfect was their top cause of stress, and around 72 percent admitted that they stressed about being stressed.

For every sunrise smoothie, yoga selfie, and "mindfulness" platitude posted on Instagram, Tumblr, Twitter, Pinterest, Snapchat, Facebook, and whatever other social platform may pop up after I type this, there's a 100 percent chance that there is a person curled up on her couch, bedheaded in sweatpants, and sick to her stomach with worry that her life will never be as lovely and serene as that.

We are legion, we anxious people. With all this technology around us, we could make noise, start visibility campaigns, go on awareness walks in matching T-shirts (though that would entail actually leaving the house . . .), write slogans, draw an adorable mascot, buy billboards, lobby for funding, anoint a celebrity spokesperson—but we don't. We suffer in silence. We hunker and hide in fear of being judged imperfect, unlovable, high maintenance, and insane. We do not speak of it.

And it is killing us by the numbers.

CHAPTER FIVE

The Horrors of Love

A few years ago, my parents pulled up stakes from their Kentucky home of nearly forty years and moved to a retirement community near my sister in South Carolina. The process took a while—a sluggish market, some home repairs, a few cold feet—and in that time, Pup gathered my childhood and shipped it to my office, box by box. I know not all parents are such dedicated curators of their children's lives; plenty or most would probably say, "Come over here and get your crap or it's going into the garbage." There was no need to clutter their pristine new home with the detritus of my life, and to be fair, I'd never asked them to keep any of it. But they did, and here it was: a portal to my past, growing in mass under my desk until I had no more room to move.

Honestly, I think it gave Pup something to do in the hours while Mumsie slept, prayed, or was prodded by doctors. While I could sense his understandable frustration, I rarely, if ever, heard him complain aloud about how things had turned out in his marriage or his life, and I've often wondered: if he knew what he was in for, the decades of caretaking, the screaming fits, the accusations, the rage, the housebound hours and seasons and years, would he have run far away? I'll never know, because he stayed and made the most of it.

And he loves her, even in the maelstrom, and maybe a little because of it. She needs, and he needs to be needed, but that's not the totality of what binds them.

She's frail and afraid now, brain and body ravaged by degenerative diseases and small strokes known as "transient ischemic attacks" that temporarily block the flow of blood to the brain, nerve damage, sciatica, fibromyalgia, rheumatoid arthritis, and seemingly constant falls that inevitably fracture her fragile bones. In her seventies, she seems ninety and he seems almost unchanged from my teenage years. She looks to him as her north. When she sees him, I think she feels the closest to safe that is possible for her.

I actually just assume this, because when Mumsie looks at me, I don't know what she thinks. I'm not always sure she makes the connection that I am her daughter. I rely on Pup's word and I let myself believe him. When I went to visit them in South Carolina for the first time, as I was leaving, I bent down to kiss her head. "I love you, Mumsie," I said, stood up, hugged Pup, and walked across the restaurant parking lot to sob in my car for a few minutes before driving back to my hotel.

He sent me an e-mail a while later: "I hope you heard her call you 'darling' when she was in the car and you were leaving, but I don't think you did hear her 'love you' as I was already closing the door when she said it. She is slow and did not get it out. EVEN MORE: when we travel she semisleeps and was doing so when we were on our way to Nan's when suddenly she said: 'Kat's pretty.' I was shocked. I cannot remember the last time I heard her give ANYONE an unsolicited, unprompted compliment. I wish you could have heard it. But you did not and I thought you should know. Feel privileged indeed. That just does not happen."

I had not heard any of this, but I chose to believe every word my father wrote. After all this time, I needed to, and Pup was kind to tell me. He's always been my north, too, even when I've been blinded by sadness and panic. And that's all I ever wanted to be for someone. From early on, I decided that even if no man could love me, because I was fundamentally flawed, I wanted to be useful and necessary, and maybe that would be enough. Not the worshiped-princess dreams of some of my friends, but I figured the fantasies were reserved for the pretty girls, the ones who knew how to flirt and bat their eyes and not talk about dinosaurs and the Brontë sisters in front of their crushes. The ones whose hands didn't shake and stomachs churn at the stupidest things. I wasn't afraid of boys—I had one as my best friend—but I wasn't at all sure how to be a girl.

In those boxes of things that Pup unearthed, amid the report cards, newspaper clippings, sad poetry, and hideous class pictures were pages from my eighth-grade diary. In addition to scintillating accounts of adolescent social politics, grumblings about teachers, and my rankings of the BEST pop groups and TV shows of ALL TIME always and forever, is a multistep plan I'd made to win the heart of my crush. It's not about pinning my skirt hem up higher, pouting prettily, riding my bike past his house, or any of the normal things a thirteen-year-old girl of the mid-1980s would do to let a boy know she liked him. It's, well . . .

Ways to Get [Name Redacted Because It's Still Too Humiliating] to Like Me:

1. Be nice to everyone.
2. Don't act crazy (i.e. screaming, laughing crazily).
3. Don't stare at him.
4. Be caring about everything.
5. My poetry, music, and art.

He is a nice person and I think that he likes caring and quiet, normal, deep people. Can I be that to him? I love him. I ask in the name of our Lord Jesus Christ, please make [redacted] ask me to go with him. Amen.

Granted, a day or two later there was an entry involving the purchase of Maybelline Kissing Slicks lip gloss and my hope that I'd get a chance to test it out on him, but otherwise the list seems almost depressingly focused on my being enough for him and not all that much of me. And definitely not, you know, crazy. Because who could love that?

My clever ploy failed. He fell for one of my infinitely more sophisticated friends (her mom sent her to modeling school and she got pictures taken and we all agreed she totally looked at least sixteen!) and I resigned myself to my lot in life as the dorky sidekick. I even helped him figure out how best to woo her. If I couldn't be happy, she might as well be.

It was Halloween soon after they connected—my favorite holiday—and I feigned sickness so I wouldn't have to see them kiss and giggle at each other all night as we made our rounds of the neighborhoods. They'd promised to stop by to see how I was feeling, and I curled up in dread in my bedroom. Shouldn't I just feel delighted that two people I liked an awful lot had found each other? Couldn't I just warm myself vicariously in their glow instead of feeling like it cast a harsh light on me? When my parents called out that it was them at the door, I wobbled up wanly, genuinely sick with upset by this point, and accepted their sympathy. Gave them extra candy, of course, to aid in their happy evening.

When I came back to school in proto-Goth mode, after my self-imposed exile/depression diagnosis, the boys I'd crushed on for as long as I could remember seemed like characters from a cartoon show I'd watched avidly as a child, but had gradually given up. Familiar in a way that was frozen in time, but that didn't have much to do with the walking, talking, learning-to-breathe-again me. The problem wasn't in their set—plenty of girls were tuned to the same channels; I just couldn't receive them. And weirdly, I didn't much care.

In many ways, it was freeing. If I didn't really give a damn what would lure these boys, seduce and entice them, I could just do what pleased me—spike up my hair, wear a studded dog collar, black lipstick, ripped tights, ragged fingernails. I was never going to be pretty in the right way anyway (at least in 1980s suburban northern Kentucky), so being relieved of that burden was an immense weight off my shoulders. Some boy wants to scream "FREEAAAAAK!" at me from a car window? Fine. I am one. I always was—but now you could see it on the outside as well. I could hang out with boys without having to fear their rejection (you can't lose if you're not playing the game in the first place) and scheme to help match up my friends for love or . . . whatever. I could bask in their happiness and pat myself on the back for all the mitzvahs I was performing without having to risk anything. Or inflict myself on anyone.

That was the thing. I was happy for them and deeply lonely. While classmates seemed utterly hell-bent on proving just how worldly they were, smoking and drinking and fooling around with wild abandon and adorable naïveté, I just watched from the other side of the glass. It was sweet and somehow pure despite their best intentions, and I didn't want to stain them with whatever toxic thing was in me and made me feel the way I did. While some of the pain and panic of anxiety had gone away because I wasn't being actively bullied every day, it had left me stranded on an island where sunlight and simple pleasures didn't often wash up. I couldn't expect anyone to meet me there.

I retreated. Physically, I sank down into my parents' basement to paint, make sculpture, write poetry, listen to music that matched my mood (lotta Cure, folks . . . lotta Cure), and generally bide my time until I could escape to college.

I'd decided to go to art school, but had panicked so badly over the prospect of being rejected, I nearly missed all my application deadlines. I'd made some new friends at the Kentucky Governor's School for the Arts between my junior and senior years in high school and they actually seemed to like me back, care about art, and join me in picking painting over parties. But I held them in awe, too. They pushed safety pins through their ears, published zines. How arrogant was I to think that I could compete with the likes of them—in college admissions or in matters of the heart? And how much was it going to hurt when they all said no?

But I got into art school—all the ones I applied to—and of course told myself that it was a fluke. I was still human—a female one to boot, and the guys who traveled with the art school kids were not to be dismissed. They weren't anything like the neatly-barbered, polo-shirted Catholic school boys I'd known since kindergarten and who barely considered me a girl anyhow. These boys wore eyeliner, dyed their hair black, painted and pinned their leather jackets with the logos of bands they loved—that I loved. Their fingers were long and slim, tipped with chipped black nail polish and guitar string calluses and if they brushed against mine, I'd shiver.

They did, weirdly, a lot of brushing against me and I couldn't quite figure out what was going on. So far as I knew from the small quantity of smut I was able to pick up at the local library or Waldenbooks (these Internet-era kids have it so much easier—and so much worse), teenage boys were ostensibly all about groping, licking, and trying to stick things in places that "nice" girls were supposed to protect. My friends, who had way more practical experience with real, live, warm-blooded, boner-having boys, would even come to me . . . definitively virginal me . . . for advice on these things (and rides to Planned Parenthood) because they knew that I was such a dork, I'd done the reading. And I also took tremendous pride in being told I had a dirty mind. My body and heart weren't getting any, but my mind was a hungry little machine, and I did my best to be useful in that regard. Blow jobs? Sure, let me look that up. Doggie style? I thiiiink I saw it mentioned in one of these Anne Rice books. I knew in theory what went where and why—I just never experienced any of it.

Chalk it up to Anne Rice being all the rage and my new penchant for vampiric flair in a boy—knife-edged cheekbones, a touch of glam, a smudge of bloody-red lipstick (his)—but my blossoming experience with boys came with a side of creepy. It kept happening, so often that if I'd been possessed of a sense of humor at the time, I'd have found it hilarious.

The boy would take an inexplicable interest in me, separate me from the herd, and I'd trot along to his car, his booth at the all-night diner, the corner of the New Wave / Goth / gay / gutter-punk club I'd begun to haunt on weekends in high school, and said boy would bite my neck, my earlobes, run his fingernails up my forearms, and lightly touch the tips of my fingers until I was a single, pulsing nerve on the verge of explosion. But he would never, ever kiss me, let alone try anything beyond that.

We'd whisper into the phone, exchange mix tapes and poems, and though I wanted more, I didn't dare ask for it. These things are meant for the girls who are not broken. The handholding, the surreptitious kisses behind open locker doors, the fogged car windows, the prom night, the possession: "Have you met my boyfriend?" These were for girls who didn't pick their skin bloody, double over sour-stomached from fear of going to the mall with their friends, whose mothers didn't scream in psychic pain then crash to sleep, who'd never stood at the edge of their world and considered doing it a favor by stepping over. They get love and you deserve scraps.

These alt-culture teenage Casanovas had girlfriends and hadn't told me, every last one of them, and in one case a fiancée. Not kissing me was their way of getting close to me but staying faithful. One is an accident, two is coincidence, and three is . . . disturbing. A pattern. An indictment from the universe. I'd been judged and found lacking, meant only as a side bit of "fun" to tease.

The first boy I got to call "mine" for a little while made me fight for him. I'd disrupted his life by showing up in it, and he let me pay for it. He'd reported for freshman year of college with the intention of being a monk, a Serious Artist, and there I was distracting him. He told me this the night he showed up to apologize for a cold shoulder earlier in the day, kissed me, annoyed, and ran away. He literally sprinted down the stairwell where we'd been sitting, out the door and into the night. He came back the next night, crawled into my slim, single dorm room bed, where I lay fevered and confused, having finally succumbed to a cold I'd been fighting off for a while. "Did I dream what happened?" I didn't even let myself say "kiss" in case I'd been hallucinating, but I needed it to be true.

I spent the whole next year with white knuckles, terrified it was going to slip away at any second, that he'd realize his mistake in choosing me, telling me he loved me, letting me share his bed. It was just a matter of time before he realized that I wasn't smart enough for him, or pretty or skinny or sophisticated, or that I got sad or panicked sometimes for reasons that I couldn't explain. There was no way I would let him see that. Certainly not that it bothered me when he would pick up a brush to "correct" my painting or wouldn't let me sleep because he wanted to see me—even when I'd been up for two days and going on three. That didn't matter because he said he loved me, and for that I owed him. And I loved him back fiercely, which is why it ground me down to dust when he ended things.

None of us could have known it then, but at the beginning of our sophomore year, he'd met the woman who more than two decades later is still his wife and is now the mother of their three children. You can't argue with a love that long-lasting—it just *is,* but at the time I saw it as a failing in me. She had to be prettier, smarter, fundamentally better than me, and I clawed myself to pieces trying to figure out what I was lacking. A mutual friend told me that my ex just felt things for her that he'd never felt before—which was not fun to hear then, and even less so in the form of a poem he read to half the school a few weeks later at an open mike. The verse praised her face and its beauty in the morning light upon waking and how he used to love me—me by name—but that it was over and I had to accept that.

That time, I ran. I bolted from the room while my best friend Beannie pulled him into a corner and swore at him (to her credit, his new girlfriend gave him hell as well; to his credit, he apologized to me eventually), and as soon as the sun rose, hopped a bus from Baltimore to my aunt's home in Pennsylvania and began the process of trying to erase myself. I knew I couldn't stay there forever, but Mumsie's twin sister, Polly, stepped in as a surrogate mother from time to time. She took me into her comfortable home, where she allowed me to cry and sleep and cry some more and brace myself to go back to a place where there had been a public declaration that I was not loved. Polly, herself, had never married or had children, but she had a lovely house and a seemingly contented life and it gave me hope that I tucked away, along with her famous home-baked choco-late cookies and the endless packets of instant soup, pasta, and tuna that she stuffed into my flimsy suitcase.

I spent the next year in Philadelphia—unable to afford a junior year abroad to somewhere exotic like many of my peers, and even less able to stomach taking five out of six classes with the ex and his girlfriend, who'd opted into both halves of the double major I'd selected. Not even my Walkman, cranked up to eleven, could drown out their happiness, so I sublet my room at school and moved to a city I'd visited only once and where I knew no one. Here's where the boundaries of my anxiety become porous. I may be utterly nause-ated by the prospect of picking up the phone, selecting a sandwich topping, or stepping out my front door, but on occasion, I can close my eyes, free-fall off the highest floor, and trust that I'll either land safely or be put out of my misery for good.

In Philly, I dropped smack into the path of Jon, who, to his credit, disclosed on our first date that before me, he'd been with a boy. "Me, too!" I cooed, delighted with myself for my open-mindedness. Two and a half years later and now living many hours apart, I was less jubilant when he told me (over the phone!) he was ending things on account of "craving man flesh." While I could take myself to task for plenty of inadequacies—it's something of a talent of mine—I couldn't exactly argue with that. Though I swore and cried an awful lot.

After him was Tony. I was in grad school by this point and giddy with the fresh, new connective power of the Internet. After meeting on an indie pop-music listserv, a few mix tapes, and a bunch of flirtatious e-mails later, I drove the six hours from the Hudson Valley to northern Virginia to see a movie with him and hopefully not get murdered. I hadn't actually seen any pictures of him before I went, but he turned out to be the prettiest boy I'd ever personally (very personally) gotten to touch up to that point. I'd have been a good amount more jubilant about that were it not for the substantial geographical miles between the two of us, not to mention the zero to hundred feet he tended to be from his recently-ex girlfriend. My worry got on his nerves, but as I learned over the course of the coming months, it wasn't unwarranted. Good-bye, pretty Tony.

Roy was plenty good and plenty kind, and I didn't want to drown him in my murk. So I bought him new clothes ostensibly for his new job, but really because I knew he'd be back out in the dating world soon. I wanted to leave him in better condition than I'd found him, so at least I wouldn't have that on my conscience. (Don't worry—Roy turned out just fine. Better than, in fact.)

Steven was just a subway ride away, but may as well have lived in a different time zone for all I saw him. Scratch that: for all I was allowed to see him. I was dazzled by him. I basked in the reflected glow of this clever man with a magazine job, fancy writer friends, Ivy League (almost) degree, New York City upbringing and tragic past. He'd dropped out of grad school—and life, essentially—to take care of his mother as she succumbed to cancer. He'd slipped under with her, and was just starting to stick a hand out above the ice when we met. I reached out to grab it.

He pulled me under with him. I don't think he knew any other way to be with another person. How could he after all that loss? I tried to give him love, but he didn't know how to take it. I assumed that meant he didn't want it. 'Cause I gotta be me.

I tried hard—too hard, by his reckoning—to be lovable, likable, interesting, witty, engaged, esoteric, cool enough for him to consider worthy. You don't want to hang out for two nights in a row because that's too much people time for you? Naw, that's fine. I'll be at home drinking this obscure single malt I bought to impress you (and which is actually pretty great . . . dammit) and reading this here impenetrable Henry James novel on a Saturday night because of course that's what I want to be doing. I'm sure this has nothing to do with the fact that you made fun of me for crying when I missed the start of *Buffy* last week and called my tastes "middlebrow." Not at all.

My anxiety is a scab that aches to be picked, and Steven and I both obliged that for two and a half years. I couldn't make him love me or accept what I offered, but he liked me enough to want to stop hurting me—and seeing me hurt myself. By the final few weeks, my worry over my worth and fear that he'd stray were so intense that my muscles locked up and I hobbled like Mumsie. He ended it. I felt the loss, of course—in our better moments we were excellent friends—but it was a mercy killing.

All I knew was that for the first time in ages I was (1.) single; (2.) not balled up with worry that the wrong words/opinion/song/restaurant/dress/poem/show was going to make him leave me. It was already done. I'd been discarded. I was lonely, but for once, I wasn't forcing myself to be alone.

I let the seams show to my friends—at first because I couldn't help it, but the more I let them in on what I was going through, the easier it became. It would have been too mortifying to admit the truth of my relationship with Steven while I was still in the thick of it. "No, I'm not running around by myself having little adventures and side projects and experimenting with different cuisines and exploring the treasures of the boroughs just because I have an insatiably curious soul and an independent spirit. It's because my boyfriend would rather not spend time with me, and when he does, I must be interesting in the exact right way."

I was now a girl going through a breakup and I didn't have to pretend that I was okay. There is a cultural precedent for that. And for when your whole department is winnowed and you're suddenly jobless. That happened, too. People understand that when you get a call that your dad's car flipped over on the highway and he's in the hospital, you probably need a hug and an escort home. Yeah, that also happened. And what's more, they don't love you any less for leaning on them. They're grateful to see you unclench a little, let your guard down, and trust them to see the real you—even if that's an anxious, needy mess.

You get a pass—for a little while—and then ideally you pry your-self off the couch, out of bed, and stand strong for the next one who needs you. I couldn't help but notice that I was standing a little taller than before. The foundation had crumbled beneath me: my partner, my family (Pup made a full recovery, but he still has glass embedded in his forearm, along with a nasty scar), my livelihood—and I didn't cease to exist. I remained in place.

And a few weeks later, when the Twin Towers were bashed out of the New York City skyline, I dug in my heels, stretched out my arms, and said, "I'm here, tell me how I can help." While all around me lay chaos, I was weirdly calm. I kept waiting to crumble, bracing for the next blow, but it never came—honestly, what more could happen?

Compared to the knee-jerk, sideswiping apps of the midtens, online dating in 2001 seems downright quaint. I'd met Steven through a dating site in 1998 and had no reason to dive back in. But now—why not? Life is, as we'd all just seen in blazing, reeking Technicolor, pretty damned short. You're still here, so go do something about it.

On nerve.com back then, pictures were optional and digital cameras were something of a novelty for personal use, so an awful lot of wooing took place in textual form.

Sam was whip-smart, sarcastic, culturally savvy, almost pinko-left in his politics, flirty, and just the right amount of dirty. Forget sexting and the tired old dick pics popping up like mushrooms on Snapchat (or so I hear from my young, single pals)—after I hungrily picked up the conversational crumbs he was scattering, our prose got a little more graphic. And I loved it. Loved wooing and being wooed with words by a man whose brain I was beginning to crave. Like Pavlov's dogs, if my e-mail pinged, my pulse quickened. I curled up with my laptop next to me in bed, sprinted home to see if he'd reached out. If a day went by (half a day, even) that I hadn't heard from him and he hadn't told me he was traveling—which he did a lot for his work as a labor activist (swooooon)—I'd curl in on myself like a plant denied sunlight.

After a few weeks, Sam wanted to speak on the phone. I froze. It's a form of communication I dread on a good day, but with my level of dependence on his contact increasing by the hour, it felt too risky, too intimate. E-mail, I could handle, take my time and craft the perfect response. But attaching an actual living person to the Sam I'd built in my head was a little too much.

I canceled the call several times before it got ridiculous, then finally admitted my worry.

"I'm afraid you'll be bored by me and I don't want to disappoint you."

"No," he said. "I just need to have your voice in my head, know that you're real."

Who was I to deny him that security?

When we finally spoke, I was stiff and strangled. This is not how I usually behaved. I talk fast, with my hands. Clamming up is not a problem I have.

But I weighed all my self-worth on that phone call. His voice eventually put me at ease, flowing into the jagged valleys, smoothing out my tension.

When we e-mailed later, Sam was warm. "Thank you for trusting me. I could tell you were nervous, but I loved your voice. I'd love to hear it in my ear before I go to sleep."

If the e-mails had been saucy—along with funny, charming, smart, and caring—the phone calls got downright filthy. He was into kink and power exchange, not excessively, but definitely as the punctuation marks in his sexual vocabulary. I was a fast learner, quickly fluent, and eager to serve. After a few years of feeling like a consolation prize in relationships, the shift from "you'll do" to "you will DO" was deeply appealing to me. I liked feeling like a sex object, even if our pleasures were only aural, and maybe because of that. If I could make a man of Sam's stature shiver with the power of my words, maybe I wasn't so intellectually challenged? And for the next few weeks we burned up the phone lines from Brooklyn to D.C., the Dominican Republic, Mexico City, Ecuador, and beyond. He was traveling constantly for work, and while we'd started to raise the specter of drinks (and maybe some of the things we'd discussed in our breathless calls) in Brooklyn, where we both lived, we just couldn't seem to get it on the books.

A few days before Christmas, he was finally going to be back in town for a day or two. Where should we meet?

I picked my favorite bar in the East Village, calculated to impress. It was a snug little upstairs room that looked out onto Stuyvesant Place and had rules. No loud talking, no groups of more than four, no standing. If the bar was full, you had to sit outside and wait, but your patience was rewarded with precisely made classic cocktails poured by solemn Japanese bartenders, and you felt awfully special.

I went out and bought a few new things: a suede, sleeveless top, a red crocodile-embossed leather skirt, and a pretty, designer-label purse. No matter what any of the exes think, you're worth it, I kept telling myself. My friend Ali kept telling me that, too, as she pep-talked me while I got ready for the date. She, more than just about anyone, had seen me through the past few boyfriends.

There was no one waiting outside the bar's door—an entrance in an alcove off a second-floor yakitori joint that was lush with sizzling grill sounds and fragrant meat. He wasn't inside either, and I told myself that if he didn't show, I could drown my sorrows in a plateful of quail eggs and skewered chicken hearts at the counter. But the truth was, I couldn't have forced any food down if I tried. It wouldn't have fit past the lump in my throat.

Five minutes passed. Then ten. Then fifteen. I stared down at the phone in my hands, fingers trembling too much to punch in the number, and when I looked up, there was Sam. Staring at me with the corner of his mouth twisted up in a smile. He didn't seem to mind what he saw either, and he told me so. "You're more beautiful in person than I'd imagined," he said.

"You're real," I said. I dropped my gaze, furiously twisted my hair in my fingers. "Shall we go in?"

We ordered our drinks: me, a sidecar, and him, a negroni, which impressed me, especially since the last date I'd taken there had ordered a cosmopolitan and kept marveling about how strong it was.

He was beautiful. In the moments when I let myself look directly at him, he took my breath away. He looked a little older than I'd imagined and definitely shorter than the five nine he'd claimed in his profile (made a note to myself: stick to flats on first dates—if there was ever another after tonight), but the Sam in my head was rapidly supplanted by the Sam sitting across from me, smiling and not looking away. And I did not mind one bit.

When I got back to the table after ducking out to tell Ali I was still alive (and totally smitten), he handed me a small box—to commemorate the moment and apologize for making me wait so long.

I opened it and gasped. This had taken time and thought. Back then, if you searched for me online, one of the things that came up was the mention of a music festival I'd emceed a few years prior, wearing long, black gloves and handing out plastic cherries with safety pins stuck through the stem so people could wear them and I could mark that I'd met them. Sam had tracked down a lovely little silver brooch shaped like a basket filled with tiny, red enameled cherries. I pinned it on right away. It matches your lips, he said, and I shivered. I was meeting the hell out of Sam.

But he kept looking at his watch and my stomach soured. I feared I was losing his interest. No, he said, I was feeling presumptuous and I made us a restaurant reservation. We should probably get a cab.

I don't remember who kissed whom first in the backseat, but I do remember the bottle of rosé Veuve Clicquot, the little jewel-box dining room where I ate real caviar for the first time, ladled with a wee mother-of-pearl spoon onto a featherlight blini lavished with crème fraîche. I ate smoked sable from his fingers—the first time any boy . . . any man had done such a thing.

"I'm swearing off utensils entirely," I told him.

"I'm so happy it's pleasing you," he said.

We got another cab, this time to my house, and once there, we did a few of the things we'd talked about over the phone. I wasn't ever this bold on a first date. But after everything I'd been through in love, wasn't it my time?

A few days later, Sam sneaked back down to Brooklyn from a family gathering in Connecticut so he could be with me on Christmas Eve, at least for a little while. I'd been thinking of driving up to Vermont to spend the holiday with my best friend and her now-husband but postponed so I could be with him.

He was amazed by me, thoroughly smitten and delighted, he said, and he showed it, too. He took me to Babbo early in the New Year and ordered Diet Coke right along with me. (Ha! Steven had begged me not to do exactly that for fear of embarrassing him.) We spent Sundays at my favorite taqueria, drank coffee while he read the paper and I babbled at him about this and that and work and life, and he never seemed to mind that Ali high-fived me when she saw what a hottie I'd bagged. His patience was beginning to wear thin in one area, however—despite all the grown-up fun we were having under the covers (and on my chaise longue, and in the shower and on the kitchen counter), we still hadn't actually had intercourse.

"I need to still have something to keep you interested," I teased . . . sort of. "If I give it all up now, you'll just be done with me."

He told me that was ridiculous, that I had plenty to offer, and hadn't he let me know that by now? But I still needed to hold a modicum of myself back, because when I go in, I go all in.

He grumbled, so I set a date, at the end of January in Las Vegas. Told him to savor the anticipation.

I arrived in town before him, was given a random upgrade to

a massive suite at the Venetian, and answered the door in my robe when Sam knocked.

Thirty minutes later, he was still interested. And an hour after that and an hour after that, and then we went to my favorite all-night restaurant for some well-earned drinks and a midnight snack. We sat in a sunken nook in the lounge, anchored by a bubbling pool of water with gas flames shooting up from the center. I snuggled into him, safe and exhausted. The waitress slinked over and, per Peppermill tradition, sat down next to us on the velveteen cushions to take our order. "Hi, I'm Candace and I'll be taking care of you two lovebirds."

I beamed. "Hi, I'm Kat!"

Sam gave a different name, and after Candace took our order, I asked him why.

"That's the thing about Vegas," he said. "You can be anyone you want to be."

I laid my cards on the table. "I can't imagine I'd want to be anyone else in the universe right now, or with anyone else either."

"Agreed," he said. And we sipped from our scorpion bowl, built for two.

The next couple of months were a blur of sex and bliss and comfort. He pushed me in my work—confident women were sexy, he said—and on the rare occasions that I had to go into the office to give a presentation or meet with my bosses, he'd advise me to wear a business suit and heels and tell him all about it afterward. He delighted in the fact that I took trips to see friends in London and sent him postcards I'd written on the plane to and from it. He made me music mixes, and when I returned the favor, he bought albums of the bands whose songs I included. He never seemed to get tired of me, even when I sobbed in frustration that he was always on the road. I'd finally found some bliss and the confidence to ask for more.

"You're needy," he said, "and I like that. I like that you need me in your life and in your bed. Sometimes I think you were built just for me."

"Sometimes," I said, "I think so, too."

Which is why I was completely blindsided when he ended things just a few weeks later. Sam showed up at my apartment, let himself in with the key I'd given him, and told me it was over. I was half-dressed, expecting him for our date, and suddenly felt more naked than I would have with no clothes on.

"Please. Why? I don't understand. What have I done?"

He was cold, matter-of-fact.

"I just don't want to. I just don't feel things for you."

The blood drained from me and I begged for my life. Am I not enough? Come to bed and I'll show you how worth it I am. Just kiss me. Just follow me. Please. Please!

He stayed the night, got dressed the next morning and went to work, and I stayed in bed, spent and terrified. I'd asked for too much.

Sam was traveling for most of the week, and on the phone, I was as blithe, obliging, and easy as I could be. No, I'm okay. Tell me all about where you are. I can't wait until Friday. I mean . . . it's cool, if you can't make it, that's cool.

He sent me an e-mail instead of showing up, afraid he would lose his will this time. Good-bye. Good luck. It's over.

Nothing made sense. I'd let him too close and he'd been disgusted with me—my panic and my neediness. I should never have cried. He saw my craziness and it must have sickened him. If he stayed with me, it would have spiraled as I declined like Mumsie, sucking him under. He must have seen that and run.

I had no idea what to do with myself. To stay in the apartment was to refresh my e-mail again and again, to see if he had updated his dating profile to say, "No paranoid, insane chicks," to listen to the songs that reminded me of him, to claw the awful thing out of me or drown it in his favorite Scotch. After a few days of that, I made a date with a friend in Manhattan, and on the way back, found myself switching trains, walking down streets as if drawn by puppet strings. In the three and a half months we'd officially been together, I'd never gone to Sam's apartment. It was messy, he told me, and he was ashamed. I understood all too well. If he were ever in town for long enough and not at my house screwing my brains out, he'd have time to clean it up, but wouldn't I rather he just spent the time with me?

I walked knock-kneed up the subway stairs toward the fruit-named streets of Brooklyn Heights. Those postcards I had sent on my way to London had to go somewhere and . . . that somewhere was a pizza shop. I stood in front of it for God knows how long, double-checking the address he'd given me, combing the block for a side entrance. There were no apartments upstairs, not a magic castle in the sky, and no evidence of a Sam Klein there or anywhere else I could find.

A message came within a few days. If you let me come by on Friday, I will explain.

The buzzer rang at the appointed time and I went downstairs to let him in. He still had his key but explained to me that he felt strange using it, and for that small bit of sensitivity, I was grateful.

When we reached my apartment, I jammed myself into the farthest corner of the chaise and wrapped my arms around a tasseled pillow to shield myself. "Talk, please."

He perched nervously at the other end, for once mindful of my space. "Everything I told you about how I feel about you is true. Please know that. Some things are not. Like where I actually live. I live in Washington, D.C."

I froze. He continued.

"And that until a couple of weeks ago, there was a wife."

The air left the room, and the light narrowed to pinpricks.

"And . . . my name."

He pulled out his weathered, much-stamped passport (at least all the travel was true) and pointed to a name I recognized—the first part at least. It was the one he'd given to Candace. The last name was one I'd never heard before.

People speak of out-of-body experiences, usually during meditation or near death. As Sam (not Sam, technically, but I couldn't wrap my head around the name of the stranger with my boyfriend's . . . someone's estranged husband's . . . face) was speaking, something inside me, perhaps my soul, detached and floated away a few feet and watched.

He was explaining that he had been married only since the previous June and maybe shouldn't have gone through with it in the first place. That she'd moved to a different state for a few months to work right after their wedding, and he'd encouraged her to do so for the sake of her career. That after 9/11, he was lonely and had gone to the dating site as a distraction and there I was and that was it—it just went too far too quickly. And that he just had to hear my voice, and then had to meet me that once, and he'd come to drinks with the intention of telling me everything, but he'd seen me and then he'd had to know what it was like to kiss me and so on.

He'd taken elaborate measures, it seemed. Bought a dedicated cell phone, took express trains and shuttle planes, stashed his ID and credit cards in a locker at Penn Station each time he was in town, paid for everything in cash. It explained why he'd told me that if I took care of the hotel in Las Vegas, he'd pay for everything else, why I couldn't find any evidence of him online, why he'd suddenly ducked down a side street one day while we were walking to the taqueria. A colleague of his was waving from across the street and seemed like she was going to come over and say hello.

He was telling me all this, he said, because he didn't want me walking around in the world thinking he'd just stopped caring about me, because he hadn't. He'd finally spilled everything to his best friend, who, after she'd told him what a monstrously sociopathic thing he'd done, told him to leave me the hell alone for the rest of my life. He told her he couldn't, that I was smart and I would figure it out, and that for once, he wanted to tell me the truth. That I'd deserved the truth the whole time.

I finally found air for words.

"Is there anything else you left out?"

"Probably, but I can't remember right now."

"Does your . . . wife know about me?"

"Yes. She found the phone bills. I think I was trying to get caught."

"Have you been sleeping with both of us?"

"No. We hadn't for months. I thought there was something wrong with me, maybe my medication, which is why I was so surprised by you and that I could."

"Medication?"

"For dysthymia—it's a low-level depression. I take a little 'holiday' from it when I come to see you so I can . . . perform."

"Are you still together?"

"We are officially separated and I spent the last week moving into my new apartment. What else do you want to know?"

I should have said, *How would you like to leave my apartment, by stairs, or by window?* or *What kind of manipulative psycho does this to another human being?* or *What gives you the right to turn me into your plaything, your mistress, without my consent?*

What I actually said was, "I'm hungry. Take me to dinner."

Think what you want to think of me, call me what you want to call me. I guarantee I have done worse to myself in the time since. I was in shock that night and for months after. At that moment, I just needed to feel sane, have some measure of the control that had been stolen from me.

A few months later, we were in bed. We'd resumed those activities again after a time, and in some ways, it was the most normal, honest communication we had. No hidden meanings or subterfuge, just a genuine meeting of bodies and hearts to a mutually gratifying end. Only, for the first time I could recall, things weren't going well. Usually deft and sure-fingered, Sam was fumbling, unable to get me where he always could. "I'm sorry," he said. "I don't know what's wrong with me today."

He'd been on a particularly vicious string of travel and was exhausted. I felt awful for him. Sam took pride in giving me pleasure and this seemed humiliating for him. "Oh, baby, don't worry," I assured him. "It's okay, let me take care of you."

And I did, and as we lay in each other's arms after, he whispered to me, "What would you say if I told you that it was all on purpose?"

"Hmmmm?" I was confused. "What was on purpose?"

He grinned at me, wriggling practically puppylike with delight. "I was playing a game, being clumsy on purpose. I wanted to see you frustrated. It excited me. Does that excite you, that I wouldn't let you come, got you right to the edge, and left you there?"

It was all I could do not to vomit on him. I wrenched as far as I could to the other side of the bed, raked my fingernails across my skin to get the feel of his hands off it. And I howled like an animal.

I had not agreed to this. I had not agreed to so many, many things with this man.

I broke.

My apartment was cold and full of him, so I hauled my laptop each weeknight, all weekend, to a nearby writing space that I could afford a little more now that I wasn't buying train and bus tickets every few weekends. Or eating in restaurants. Or at home. Or participating in life in any real way. I stayed in my hole writing pages upon pages of a chick-lit novel in which girl meets boy who isn't who he seems and boy turns out to be someone even better. (That book is 120,000 words long, has never been read by anyone, and it may be best if it stays that way.)

The heft of that book kept me tethered to the earth. So did the pills I started taking for the first time in a decade and a half. I held out as long as I possibly could, utterly terrified and repulsed by the deadening effect they seemed to have on my mother's whole being, but it hurt too much to be in my skin. The worry and sadness were burning holes in me, and I imagined people could see straight through to my punctured heart.

I was given a low dose of Effexor XR, a combination antidepressant and antianxiety drug that I now believe to be Satan in capsule form (we'll get to that later). It did jack-all for the latter and I still woke up every morning on the floor of the Arctic Ocean, but at least there was a small bit of sleep to be had. And for the first time in a while—actually, ever—for the first time ever in my life, my immediate reaction to stress wasn't a roiling stomach and the taste of my most recent meal in the back of my throat. It wasn't that I stopped being upset or worried—it was just that there was suddenly a buffer between my screeching hyena mind and my nervous system, and I could spare an extra second or two of rational thought about how to deal with the situation at hand rather than flailing about for whatever would mollify it most quickly.

This was progress. This is what kept me from upending my mai tai onto a man's head when, on our third date, he berated me for not letting him finger me in the back room of an East Village bar, and then told me, Listen . . . I know I told you my name was Eric, but it's really . . .

I stopped listening. The blood thrumming in my ears drowned out his voice. It didn't even occur to me to actually be angry with him, because this was apparently just the way I was to be treated. I'd taken a chance, stuck a pinkie toe back into the dating pool after a few months, and, well, I should have just expected that. There must have been a memo I'd missed—the one where I'd officially been labeled as "damaged goods"—so I decided to shelve myself for a while.

And I let Mistress Cherry take my place.

IRRATIONAL FEAR #3
SEEING THE DOCTOR

I am a trapped and terrified rabbit and if I could play dead I would. My pulse betrays me, though, so I just have to wish behind crushed eyelids and locked knuckles that it will be over soon.

It's my fault. I knew that even before the paper-masked dentist started muttering over and over that it wouldn't be so bad if I had just come in sooner, but I'm not in any position to express my agreement. I just need not to be in my body right now and attempt to astrally project to somewhere more pleasant: a beach, a bar, the middle seat between two screaming toddlers on a transatlantic red-eye—just anywhere I don't have to have my jaw ratcheted open and crammed with several dozen gloved fingers, a rusty garden trowel, wet cardboard, and a chain saw. Oh God, are those wet, flying flecks just chunks of my teeth that she's grinding off? I should have left the second I saw the intake form with __ / __ / 19__ as the date field, but I didn't because I grew up Catholic, and if nothing else, we are hell-bent on paying penance for all transgressions.

Bless me, Doctor, for I have sinned. It's been about two decades since my last appointment. I beg for thy mercy for I have flossed like a mofo in the interim.

She shows me none, and neither does the ice-faced hygienist who entered the room twenty minutes earlier to heave a leaded apron onto me, shove bulky, knife-edged objects against my inner cheeks, and bark the words "BITE!" and "RELEASE!" at me until I raise my paws in surrender. I suspected from her accent that those were the only words of my language she knew, and I was bereft of any in hers—or my own, by that point, so soft, terrified sobs would have to do.

The dentist keeps drilling. Why would anyone wait so long? Let their gums bleed and a gray line etch itself across the top of their tooth—why would anyone?

I don't claim to know anyone's anything, only mine and barely that. After the last time I'd gone to the dentist, still in grad school and swaddled in the accompanying health care plan, I got broke for a while. Not poor—poor is so much harder to come back from. I was broke because I had enough, and then I didn't for a while. I was sure that since I'd had enough at one point, I'd have enough again, and since I'd grown up with doctors and dentists and check-ups and fluoride rinses and braces—maybe it would be okay to let the professional-dental-care thing slide for a while as I figured out how to keep a roof over my head and ignore my stomach rumbles. Pup sent me vitamins in the mail because Mumsie made him, I think. "I'm fine" was a lie I needed to tell all of us.

When I did finally find a job with actual benefits—not just my cobbled-together collection of tasks and hours and sealed enve-lopes of cash (the art biz is weird, man), it just seemed like a waste to go to doctors, save for birth control. And even that went poorly. Hours after a condom ruptured, I hightailed it to the offices of the woman I'd designated as my primary care physician (without ever having met her). Before deigning to dole out the launch codes to deploy the high-test progestin pills as a morning-after solution, she took me to task for not having already been on The Pill. Called me reckless and careless as I explained through teeth gritted to keep from chattering that pregnancy was perhaps my single greatest fear, and if I'd had one single extra cent to spend on something that wasn't Top Ramen and subway fares to work while I was uninsured, I would have gone that route, but here we are. I apologized over and over, as if I'd done something to sully her body, not mine, because you defer to doctors and don't push back. I swallowed the first round and heaved up my sandwich in the restroom of a cheap, smug vegetarian restaurant a few blocks from her office. I'm sorry. I'm sorry.

After that, save for the occasional unsolvable-by-Theraflu-or-Pepto issue, I avoided physicians' offices like a man-made plague unless my annual birth control prescription re-up necessitated it. Therapy was one thing—I'm a person who needs that as much as air, noodles, and sunshine to thrive, and it'll likely be that way as long as I have the means to do it and a sentient human licensed to put up with me. But the thought of another exam where I'd sit shivering in a paper gown while being berated for insufficient self-care seemed counterproductive at the least. Patronizing and invasive at the most. I took the birth control speech to heart and spent the next several years attempting to convince my next doctor to help me with a more permanent solution than a pill, but she (and the Catholic-backed hospital for which she worked) refused to even entertain the notion. You're too young. You don't know what you want. You'll change your mind. Good luck finding a husband with an attitude like that, and by the way, we told the pharmacist you can't have your current prescription filled until you get that chlamydia cleared up.

Say . . . what? I'd been slightly baffled when the pharmacist told me to call my doctor and I spent a solid two hours with my stomach in my throat until I could get ahold of her to explain. You know . . . your chlamydia? The hell I did—I was single and before that had been in a relationship for two and a half years. This would have meant he'd cheated. This would have meant I'd been walking around with it for the year since I'd last been in her office. This would have meant . . .

This actually meant that she hadn't bothered to check my chart before roadblocking my prescription. She vaguely remembered I'd been in for something (it was a UTI, for the record) and decided just to go with a chlamydia verdict over the phone because she hadn't felt like walking back to the record room to double-check my file. It was as good an excuse as any not to go to her—or any doctor, if I could possibly manage it.

Because if you don't go to the doctor, they can't tell you that you're sick in a way that can't be fixed.

And the longer you go between visits, the harder it is to come back. When was your last physical, flu shot, Pap smear, tooth cleaning, eye exam, cholesterol test, mammogram, mole check—all these things that reasonable adults are supposed to have mastered? Once I met Douglas, I was a top-notch nag about these things (not so much the Pap smear and mammogram), because if I couldn't do this for myself, I could give a double-sized damn about the health of the man I was marrying. (For his fortieth birthday/our engagement party, I had the guests all scream, "Go to the damn doctor!" at him when he rounded the corner, such was my fervor on the subject. I was just shy of thirty-four and feeling creaky, but immortal.)

Your brain can lie all you let it, but your body eventually tells the truth. My breasts started hurting differently than they ever had during a menstrual cycle. That, I was used to—a dull ache. This was sharp and in strange places and there's breast cancer in my family, and that fear outweighed the others. It became a cannonball when the (new) doctor's office left a voice mail about "abnormal mammogram results" at 4:55 on a Friday afternoon and I couldn't reach anyone until Monday, and an entire battalion's artillery when the radiologist said "Hmm . . ." during the second round and ultrasound a few days later. It metastasized into rage when I called my doctor's office to explain the strange letter I received from the department of health a couple of weeks later informing me that I had "dense breasts" and should have my health care provider explain. (This is actually a letter you get in the mail if you have these particular test results in New York State. Presumably a strip-o-gram was out of their price range.) They'd received the test results, too, and just hadn't thought to let me know—or explain them in an especially useful fashion. "They're just . . . dense. Like, the tissue is dense."

I still don't know if I'm ashamed of or proud of myself for not snotting back, "I know you are, but what are my tits?!" but I kept my composure as best I could while she went on to explain that I'm just lousy with cysts and that I'll have to deal with them from time to time. And that for me, regular care and screenings aren't optional. Rock crushes scissors. Scissors cut paper. Paper with scary threat of cancer smothers fear of motherlike diagnosis. I go to a doctor now. She's really nice and e-mails me right back and has great Yelp reviews.

But the dentist. I'm mortified to say it was vanity that finally drove me into the chair—the aforementioned gray mark darkening into something I could no longer tell myself was a coffee stain. I was going to lose a tooth—a highly visible one—and it was all my fault. The world would know (at least until I could get a fake one installed) that I was such a careless, cowardly person that I deserved to be defanged. And the pain, too. Over the previous months, I'd developed a daytime molar-grinding habit that had begun to cause head and neck aches—because the anxiety demons had decided my thumb skin I constantly clawed and stomach lining weren't quite enough to feed them.

So I book an appointment at the closest office to my apartment that accepts my insurance. Whatever fate deals me, I will accept. Even when the (albeit tidy and functional) office decor looks like it hasn't been updated since the early 1990s. Even when half the pamphlets in the racks are in what appears to be Cyrillic, from a culture not known for its gentle or cutting-edge oral surgery. Even when the hygienist shoves an object in place so roughly I taste blood. And even when the dentist enters and the machines whine and I'm fairly certain my soul is leaving my body, sucked out wetly by a yellowed spit tube nestled against the bottom of my gums.

One of the unexpected benefits of being scared of everything is that very few of these things turn out to be as awful as you imagine they will be. They just can't be or none of us would ever leave the house. But at this moment, that seems like a highly prudent trade-off—forgoing restaurants and friends and movie popcorn and sunshine in exchange for not being pinned to this chair. The doctor is doing her best to soothe (and I am mortified that my distress is that obvious), but this is perhaps not her forte. It's only this bad because you waited so long . . . I still don't understand why twenty years . . . next time will be easier, but you gave us so much we have to do first . . .

I feel the machine whir and pierce through a space between my bottom front teeth that wasn't there before, and a shard of something catch my tongue. A tool moving, electric against the gum between my teeth where the hole is now. Even with my eyes squeezed shut, I know my vision has gone gray.

When the machines slump to sleep and my mind drifts back into my fear-spent body, I'm blurry. Not everything has snapped back into alignment, but she hands me a mirror. The gray line has been scraped away and my eyetooth saved from the dental gods. They took something else, though, as their toll.

She's telling me I'm lucky. That most people would have been left with a mouth of crumbs after so much neglect (seriously, I brushed and flossed like it was my damn job, people), but I'd been spared because of excellent genetics. Now the woman at the front desk can schedule my next appointment for a night guard and a deep cleaning, once they're approved by my insurance company, but when the appointed hour arrives, I can't make myself leave my desk. I can't answer the phone when the office calls. I just bolt down the rabbit hole and wish for luck.

CHAPTER SIX

In the Dungeon

Have you ever in your adult life slapped another grown person full across the face? If you're both on board with that happening, it can be remarkably cathartic and strangely calming. An order is established, pain meted out and accepted, and it's such a shock to both your systems that you earn a temporary reprieve from reality.

In the wake of Sam's deceit, clearly neither my head nor my body could be trusted to get an accurate read on anyone's intentions. If something so basic as a name could be a lie, why should I bother trying to live by mine?

So, I gave myself a new one: Mistress Cherry.

My alter ego was better suited to living in the world, as Kat Kinsman clearly wasn't doing a bang-up job of it. I wandered around listlessly, afraid to give a damn about anything in case it turned out to be a lie. I'd tried dating a little online but ghosted away when the possibility of an in-person meeting reared its head. There's only one way this ever ends for me. I threw myself into work, crawled under the covers when it was done, and met each morning with a flinch. Who's going to hurt me today? Does everyone know what a weak, pathetic fool I have been? There's the girl who's so naive she didn't even know her own boyfriend's name.

A friend had managed to pry me from my apartment one night, insisting that it would be healthy for me to be around other people. While I was formulating my escape plan from the bar, another acquaintance mentioned that a friend of hers had just recently taken a job as a professional dominatrix. She was working in an S&M dungeon in Manhattan. For the first time in months, my interest in something other than sleeping, crying, and obsessively Googling was piqued.

Days later, I was cinched into a corset and some cruelly high boots, attempting to summon the courage to slap a stranger across the face. It's not a thing that comes naturally to most of us, willfully harming another human being, and especially not outside the heat of anger. With a cool head, most rational human beings would not lift their palm, haul it back for maximum velocity, and make contact with a naked cheek.

My head was not especially cool that first afternoon in my new role. It was a couple of weeks before Thanksgiving and the sun was already being swallowed up by the night sky at what seemed like noon every day. In a good year, I'm not the hugest fan of the holidays—the expectation of being shiny and bright tends to sharply contrast with my circumstances. I was at my coldest, lowest, brokest, loneliest, and the hordes of holiday revelers inevitably set me off.

Yes, I'm happy you're here in my city to see the giant tree, the Rockettes, Santa at Macy's, the lights, the dazzle, the miracles—I'm just trying to get a seltzer and an egg sandwich and not terrify anyone with my hollow-eyed stare.

I'd muscled my way through cars and crowds walking from my therapist's office, feeling more defeated with each step. I slipped on a slush pile scooting out of the way of some tourists on a narrow West Village sidewalk and braced my fall to the wet concrete with my knee and palms. I stayed there for a minute on the ground, umbrella twisted beneath me and soaked to the skin, too humiliated to move.

I limped gingerly the rest of the way, still shaking and damp as I ascended the stairs to the loft for my training session. I'd dabbled in kink with a few boyfriends—one who liked to cross-dress, another into bondage, and of course with Sam, when he bothered to tell me beforehand what was happening—and it made me feel special. Even if I couldn't be pretty and sexy in a way that most of the world understood, I knew at a gut level how to play this role. I had a few friends into the burlesque scene, and at an annual festival, a clothing vendor enticed me into trying on a tight-laced corset to go with a saucy candy-striper ensemble. Standing up tall, hard and slick in shiny PVC, I looked invincible.

But now, who was I kidding to think that anyone would see this wreck of a girl—surely they would peer through the kinky costume—and wish for her to assume dominion over them? Certainly not Jakob, the training slave who served the dungeon by letting the new girls learn their craft by using his skin as a canvas. He'd seen it all, and had his routine down.

"Cut my nipple off, I beg of you," he said as the headmistress led me into the red-bricked front room where I'd had my interview the weekend before. It was tidy, save for the long black coat, white dress shirt, hat, and tzitzit Jakob had heaped on a black-cushioned bench, and the walls were lined with all manner of pain-bringing instruments, from floggers and paddles to slim, sharp canes and single-tailed whips.

"Clean that up," she barked at him. "And ignore him," she told me. "He says that to everyone."

"Oh," I thought. "Perhaps I can just pretend I have an appointment I forgot about and slip out now. This was a mistake. I need to leave with my dignity and psyche intact, because—"

"Good job, Jakob. You two have fun now!" The headmistress clomped out of the room on her thick-soled, spike-sided boots and I was left staring at this small, fuzzy, undershirted man who I was supposed to learn to harm.

"Please, please cut my nipple off, Mistress!"

"Uhhhh . . . no thank you."

"My cock?"

"Yeah . . . NO."

"Then will you at least please do me the tremendous pleasure of slapping me in the face?"

This seemed benign by comparison—amputation versus a thing that little girls on playgrounds do—and yet I was still having trouble raising my hand to strike this man in front of me. This isn't what good girls do. What nice girls do. What I do. But then again, where had being nice and good gotten me? I could be my sweetest and kindest, give everything to a man and muffle my own desires, and still be tossed aside in a moment. Perhaps I should give inflicting pain a try.

"Please, please, Mistress. You would be doing me a kindness."

That did it. I hauled back my hand, cracked it across his cheek so hard his glasses flew off, and in the shock of the moment, I drew the back of my hand against the other side of his face upon the return.

He gasped, recovering his breath and curling to the floor to retrieve his glasses, tuck them atop the pile of his clothing for safe-keeping. "Thank you, Mistress. That was perfect."

I, on the other hand, was breathing deeply and easily for the first time in recent memory—certainly since Sam. We'd played around, but never with physical violence and certainly not with me calling the shots. Our games involved words and postures, perhaps a small bit of restraint. He'd left a mark on me, to be sure, but never a visible one like the handprint quickly reddening Jakob's face. I was calm. I was in control. This was a gift.

"Mistress, I humbly ask because I was not told—is there a name you would wish for me to call you?"

I paused for a moment, took a slow breath, and gathered my thoughts while he waited. In the wake of Sam, I'd stopped feeding myself, added more tattoos to slip out of the naked skin he'd touched. My most recent addition was a pair of ripe, red cherries etched into the left side of my upper back.

"When I allow you to speak, you may call me Mistress Cherry. I will never remove anything from you, not a nipple and certainly not your cock. If you please me, after a while, I may give you something, a scar perhaps. But now you are going to show me how to give you pain."

I reached for a flogger made with strands of ball bearings, and through his screams, Jakob thanked me over and over again. From there, I was thrown into the fray. I made it up as I went along, relying on my gut, empathy, and memories of old Anne Rice books to get me through each session.

I buried myself in Mistress Cherry. She was the demon who had been living inside my head since the boys in high school bit and scratched but never kissed me—all teeth and nails and spit and whips, no tenderness. She could say and do all the things I couldn't and men would crave her attention, pay her for the privilege of being in her presence and injured by her. The dungeon had some hard, fast rules, and Cherry's were even more stringent in order to protect the soft strands of myself that were still inside.

The dungeon was a technically legal enterprise: no sex or "jobs" of any kind, you never accepted cash directly from a client, tips were split evenly with the house, you kept all surfaces and all implements almost surgically clean, you showed up for your shifts on time, and you constantly maintained your training.

Mistress Cherry allowed no one to touch her during a session, save for a pedicure if she especially felt like indulging an obedient foot slave. She allowed no sessions that mimicked intercourse (which knocked her out of the running for most of the clients, who were pretty much straight dudes too scared to ask their partners to strap on an implement and do them in the ass). No Roman, brown, or ruby showers (you can go ahead and Google those if you wish to, but I do not recommend it), and nothing that bored her or made her feel unsafe.

She needed . . . I needed to stay in total control.

It started with my body, drawn and squeezed into leather and PVC corsets to mold my waist, hips, and tits into a cartoon hourglass—inhuman proportions achieved through pain. Having a colleague pull the laces tight with their hands wasn't nearly enough. Exhale, grab on to something solid, and brace for the foot in the center of my back so the cinch could be stronger. I'm not there until I see stars. Then more laces and buckles on thick-soled and high-heeled boots over seam-backed stockings. Blunt-cut bangs, red lipstick, vinyl gloves up past the elbow unless my claws needed to come out, which they often did. There's a particular art to being naked and clad at the same time, and I mastered it.

What you could enlist Cherry to do was personal, lovingly delivered pain. Say you were a twentysomething Orthodox Jewish man who had not felt truly cared for since his father had passed away. She would tenderly arrange your trembling body on a kneeling bench with your face turned to the side to observe the proceedings in the mirror. She would chastise you for your failings in class, your barely adequate grades, the shame you brought upon the family, your laziness. And she would spank you, skillfully and deliberately, as your body released and you wept with pain and gratitude. Or perhaps you were a very odd fiftyish man who needed chunks of ice whipped at you and a particular brand of spearmint gum chewed near your ear while your mother berated you for having listened to your baseball game on the radio rather than doing the laundry for the mental ward where she, the head warden, was raising you. Cherry wasn't there to judge.

Or there was the man who needed his chest knelt on and a stainless-steel dental gag ratcheted open when he failed to deliver the launch codes in the spy scenario he'd scripted. Or the man whose lifelong dream was to be consumed alive by a giantess (he was turned into an elaborate human sundae on one occasion, mummified in slices of mortadella atop a bed of greens on another, and turned into a tropical fruit salad in the center of a kiddie pool on another). Or the one who needed to be spit and stepped on, kicked hard in his most tender spots, then told sweetly, softly in his ear how worthless, low, and needy he was that he had to resort to such a thing—and that Cherry cared for him and was helping to correct him by laying out his flaws for all to hear.

I'd dissolve into a fugue state during these sessions, especially when verbal abuse and small, intense damage was required—a pinch, a flick, a scratch, a bite. When I'd return to consciousness, if another of the girls was in the room observing or taking part, I'd inevitably find her gape-mouthed and dizzied by the intimate, specific cruelty Cherry had delivered. "You're terrifying. Where does that come from? I could never do that." These women could deliver an elegant, nicking lash of a single tail, bury themselves elbow-deep in someone's ass, and hang a human being from ceiling hooks, but my words somehow sank even deeper through the skin.

So far as I understand, the world of commercial dungeons has changed—at least in NYC. The one where I worked has since been raided and dismantled (after I left, it would seem that not all of the newer girls had gotten the "no jobs" memo), and it's up to independent practitioners to tend to the city's kinky clientele—who are, by the way, just normal human beings who you'd never suspect enjoy being whipped, electrocuted, or dressed up like a pretty prom queen. They're CEOs, law enforcers, accountants, teachers, athletes who all just have an itch that's a little trickier to reach. I did my damnedest to make them feel safe, unashamed, and heard, and if I knew they had a partner, I encouraged and coached them to bring up the subject so they could explore it in the safety (and with considerably smaller expense) of a relationship. Just because I was going to die alone and emotionally scarred didn't mean everyone else had to.

And from the clients, all men, I was met with nothing but gratitude and a constant refrain: thank you for understanding me, for not judging, for not calling me a weirdo, for freeing me from myself for a little while. I needed to maintain the facade—after all, that was what they were paying me for—but I was equally grateful to them for their trust and their honesty. There may be games aplenty in a dungeon, roles, costumes, and scripts, but it takes guts to show your freakish needs to another person, and I appreciated the bravery every single time. I also welcomed the inevitable hug I was given at the close of the session (after they'd showered and dressed, of course, because EEW!). It was only then that they were allowed to touch me, and I'd assess each time if it was Cherry or me sending them out into the world with that embrace. Some needed to feel the surge from an avenging bitch goddess who they could rely on to wrest them from their mortal life when they needed, and others—just plain sweetness. Good-bye, good luck, and you're welcome.

The hugs were really the only physical human contact I was allowing myself at this time. While Mistress Cherry was vinyl-skinned and steel-hearted, I was still tender and bruised, descending to street level from my fifth-floor walk-up only when absolutely required. The Effexor I had started taking helped blunt the impact of contact a little bit, and swiftly, it had twined onto my nervous system, making it utterly dependent.

But the dungeon helped, too, the adrenaline and endorphin blasts of an excellent session balancing out the deficit I'd been feeling since Sam had scraped me hollow. I fantasized about him finding out how I'd rebuilt myself. Cherry's on top now, and you may not have a taste.

Looking back, I can see I was crafting a hard cast around me so all the broken parts could heal. I'd given everything I had to Sam and he'd taken the rest from me—my trust, dignity, sense of safety and balance. It's devastating enough to weather a breakup, going through the emotional rewiring afterward, so they're not the first person you think to reach out to when something wonderful or horrible happens, so you remember in your half sleep not to reach out, because their head is no longer on the other pillow, so you know they're not the reason your phone just lit up. I'd had to accept that I'd never actually known who that other person was. That even when I gave him a second chance to tell me (and convinced all my friends—who wanted to maim him—that they should as well), I wasn't worth much more than some rowdy sex and a few dinners out. Gonna treat me like a whore? I guess I'll act like one—or at least as close as I could stomach.

I stripped down my life, made it unfamiliar so there were far fewer chances for me to stop and ache for that naive girl who'd gotten hurt, and so no one I knew could ask me how I was doing. I had new, outrageous stories to tell ("This one regular likes to have these slim, metal rods called sounds shoved up his . . .") and they drowned out all other sound—even if not all my friends really wanted to listen. Oh, I was unbearable, I'm sure, but I didn't have it in me to care. They're great tales to tell at parties, and I appreciated the opportunity to be the loudly desired girl (paid, even!), and note the occasional looks of judgment and disgust from my friends, more than having yet another person come up to me with gritted teeth and pity in their eyes. I heard what happened to you. Are you doing okay?

Honestly, I wasn't sure what "okay" was and if it would ever mean for me in a romantic sense what it did for other people. It was almost a relief. I was good at this new way of being with men: I hurt and humiliated them and they thanked me, and they had no power to harm me, inside or out. Hell, they didn't even know my real name. If I could give up the worry of being a real, human, romantic woman who wondered what the man in front of her actually wanted, I'd be freed up to spend the rest of my energy on my friends (at least the ones who weren't totally sick of my gnarly tales) and work (my clients had no idea their websites were being built and managed from the employee lounge of a dungeon), and that would be enough, I decided. I had a friend in London who I had slept with from time to time over the years, with great affection and no particular drama attached, so if we could keep up that arrangement, maybe I could go ahead and cross romantic angst off my worry list for the rest of time. Okay, excellent plan!

The other unexpected benefit of my strange sideline was that it actually got me out of my apartment and out into the world on a regular basis—maybe not the normal world so much, but at least not hunched up sobbing in my bed and watching *West Wing* DVDs until 5 A.M. While my interactions with humanity within the confines of the dungeon might have been outside the standard social contract, they made a particularly interesting framework for the rest of humanity—and a calming one at that. Website client being difficult? Imagine them handcuffed onto a rack awaiting the next lash of your flogger. Fellow commuter won't shut up? Picture them muffled by a ball gag. I didn't wish anyone harm (at least not that they didn't request), but the notion that I potentially had some measure of control in my own life—that no person and no swinging serotonin levels could strip from me—was what I needed to cling to.

If a problem came along, Cherry could whip it real good. So I let her.

IRRATIONAL FEAR #4
TALKING ON THE TELEPHONE

Few things can send me into a terror spiral more quickly than a ringing phone—or nowadays, a Facetime request (not while I have my curlers in!)—when I'm not prepared for it. In ye olden days before caller ID and even answering machines, the only way to end the torment was to pick up the clanging beast and see who was making the intrusion into your day. In my mind, clearly it means that someone has died, needs bail money, or is hiding in the house, taunting me before slaying both me and the adorable children I am babysitting. Either that or my alma mater wants money. But it's never good.

I'll stare at the ringing phone—and Google the number if need be—with a suddenly quickened pulse, convinced that the caller can see me and judge me for my hesitation. "I'll call them back," I tell myself. "Or send a text. Maybe an e-mail. Or flowers—everyone likes flowers. I'll do that. 'Dear So-and-So, sorry I missed your call, I was going into a tunnel. Here are some Gerbera daisies as an apology for your having to deal with having such a pathetic friend.'" That may sound like an exaggeration, but I have at least two 1–800-Flowers receipts to prove it. (And of course I placed the orders online.)

I didn't always loathe the phone—in the less complicated days of childhood, few things made me happier than chatting with friends across town or down the street about which boys were cute, who was squabbling with whom, and how much homework plain ol' sucked. The landline was a lifeline to a house less fraught than mine, and I could crawl through it to safety for minutes, hours at a time.

And then one day, it was snipped. Elle sneaked Lana on to a spare receiver and told me she had said terrible things about me. It was a Sun Tzu–level bullying tactic designed to elicit nasty words from me about Lana, so Elle could prove to her that I wasn't a loyal friend. I didn't take the bait—I just whimpered, wounded, until they both came on the line and Elle dressed me down for being such a weak person as to believe what she'd told me. (Warlords have nothing on middle school girls.) That was one million years ago, and still, some small part of me wonders if another party with my best interests far from the center of their heart is listening in, and I find myself being guarded with my words whenever I'm on the phone.

And then there were the calls of duty, from which I'd unsuccessfully try to hide. When I was growing up, my mother's family expected a phone call from her (us) at some point on Sunday afternoon. I'd do my best to be unavailable at the time and avoid having to get grilled en masse by her parents and siblings who'd all perched on their extensions in various parts of my grandparents' home in Pennsylvania. "How is your figure?" my grandmother would inevitably start. (Uhhh . . . fine? Holding steady at a 32A, but here's hoping!) Grades. Sports. Extracurriculars. Tick off the accomplishments for the week, okay, you're dismissed—until the point in my life at which they decided I was weird and destined for failure.

"You're still serious about being an artist? Don't come crying to us when you're in the poorhouse. Get a teaching degree as backup for when you come to your senses." "Is your hair still that color is was in the picture your mom sent? When are you going to look normal again?"

I did my best to remain neutral or invisible, but learned a steady dread of the phone—especially after the year when Mumsie decided that Christmas afternoon was the perfect time, with the family all assembled in the spirit of Yuletide cheer and virgin births, to let them know how they'd failed her and how it had affected her faith in God. I managed to stitch together enough of the shrieks and sobs to figure out that her therapist had suggested this course of action, but in a letter. One that was not to be mailed. Thanks, Santa.

The phone is awkward, and I get performance anxiety when I'm forced to use it. There are no facial expressions to read or gestures to augment an awkward silence. (Yes, yes, Facetime, Skype—I find them even more invasive and awkward and pretty much have them blocked from my life.) I would rather board a plane, TSA pat-down included, sit with a person for several hours, and fly back home than hop on the phone for a little catch-up chat where inevitably I feel as if I'm being insufficiently entertaining. I live in terror of small talk and inevitably start to babble just to fill the silence. Then after I hang up, I revisit the conversation in my head in red-faced horror at the stupid things I must have said.

I like e-mail. Endlessly editable e-mail. (And my figure is just fine, thank you. Merry Christmas.)

CHAPTER SEVEN

Drifting, Falling, Landing

Even a rough, tough, leather-clad hell vixen (or someone doing her best to role-play at being one) needs a little softness in her life. Mine came in the form of a trembling little black-and-white rescue bunny I renamed Claudette. She'd been called "Bugsy" when I met her because of the way her kohl-rimmed eyes bugged out from her head when she was terrified. In fact, the head of the rescue group attempted to dissuade me from selecting her, telling me that she wasn't a suitable pet for a first-time rabbit owner.

"Poor Bugsy here was stuck in a cage with a little boy who used to try to spook her and poke at her with sticks. Then he got bored because she wasn't 'fun' enough and just sat in the corner and shook. See how her eyes bug out? That's why. Stupid parents just didn't want to take care of her anymore, which is why she's here, and she's been here probably two years. She'll probably always be here. People want emotional validation from a pet, and Bugsy's not the girl for that. No one wants a bunny that's just scared and hides all the time."

Oh, lady, little do you know. In a penned-off hallway, Claudette hopped right over to me, rubbed her chin and scent glands on my shoes to mark me as hers, and I knew better than to argue. It was the most honest display of affection and trust I'd received in ages, and a year and a half after Sam's final exit, I was finally ready to let another heart beat in my home. You and me against the world, little bunny. Let's take care of each other.

I don't know if it was Mistress Cherry or Kat who decided on the first day of 2005 to stride back into the online dating world (who knows—maybe it was Claudette?). I actually do know. It had to be Cherry, because Kat would never in a million years have written such a saucy, confident, devil-may-care ad. Kat would have tortured herself over every line, doubted the validity of the enterprise, and decided to abandon the exercise halfway through. I was at peace with my romantic solitude—love just wasn't in the cards for me, and that was okay. Right? I loved my friends (who were frankly getting sick of my often graphic stories and just wanted to hang out without having the discussion turn to bodily fluids and sharp objects), had an actual job (other than the dungeon) that paid decently and allowed me the freedom to be wherever I needed to be (usually on my laptop, in my bed, sometimes from the dungeon). I had my bunny. So what if I'm alone forever? It's better than the sick, sad thing I'd mistaken for love before. Right? Right?

Wrong. Life is both excruciatingly long and punishingly short (and my ass and chest were only going to stay this perky for so long), and I could press the ejector button at any point, now that I'd seen I could survive alone in space. After spending New Year's Eve kissless at the home of two newlywed friends, between Cherry and me, one of us hit the publish button.

It seemed there were an awful lot of single souls looking to start the New Year off with a bang. The ones who just wished for fleshy fireworks, I simply deleted. Poor punctuation, sloppy spelling? Fizzle. I bantered back and forth with a few and then, on the morning of January 6, burst out laughing.

Part of the ad I'd placed read like so:

More About What I Am Looking For:

You are kind. Oh, goodness, you are kind. You're also brilliant, hilarious, adored by your friends, passionate, and memorable.

You know the difference between "your" & "you're" and "it's" & "its" and it drives you nuts when people confuse them. You'd never even dream of pluralizing with an apostrophe.

You don't spit in public or think of sweatpants as potential dinner wear. You also shower. Frequently. With soap, even.

You're nice to the waiter and tip well.

You're not afraid to melt for me sometimes.

You've got a big, nasty brain and you're not shy about using it.

You know what you're doing in the kitchen, the bedroom, and the library, and ideally do NOT own a Nintendo, PlayStation, or whatever machine the kids are into these days.

You think a good blend of autonomy and affectionate solidarity seems pretty ideal.

And a man named "StoneRaven" had responded, in part:

I don't own sweat pants (just those two words together are gross—sort of like "moist slacks"). What if the two words together were verb / object . . . could one actually sweat pants? Would it hurt?

I couldn't honestly say, but I needed to find out more about this man. And I did over the next ten days. He was a North Carolina native, six years older than me, claimed to have actual friends with whom he seemed to spend a good deal of time, owned two dogs, had a hell of a great sense of humor, and a creative streak a mile wide.

He didn't seem to give a damn that I had a side gig slapping men around. I'd mentioned it almost as a deterrent—a warning that if you can't deal with all the different parts of me, you just plain old don't get access to any of it. Not that I was especially convinced that he wanted access, but I had to try . . . didn't I? While he noted that it wasn't his particular proclivity and that he wasn't himself a fetishist of any kind (beyond appreciating a really great bottle of Bordeaux), he liked that I was confident enough to know myself and not apologize for it.

Was that true? I wasn't sure, but apparently I was playing it effectively online. Might as well go all in. My dungeon comrades and I were booked as hostesses of a fetish night at a club on the Lower East Side and I double-dog-dared him to show up. I told him it was five dollars if you show up in fetish gear, seven if you came wearing some interesting fabric like leather or PVC, and ten if you showed up in regular clothes. And that it didn't start until ten o'clock, which might be past his bedtime on a Sunday night.

He said he'd be there.

I was running late—partially because it takes an awfully long time for half a dozen dominatrices to get everything properly cinched and buckled, and partially because I was terrified that he wasn't going to be there . . . or that he was.

So when I strode into the bustling, darkened bar in knee-high, cloven-soled, red-pony-fur boots, with a hedge-fund manager in a tutu and fairy wings on a leash by my side, I was doing my level best to remain in charge of my demeanor. Head up, shoulders back, eyes steeled and scanning the crowd. I'd seen a few pictures, but you can never quite tell what someone looks like in real life, in the flesh.

Not him. Could be him? Definitely not him. And then I yanked my little pet's chain and strode over to the tall man in the leather pants, white shirt, and black cowboy hat leaning up against the bar, observing the proceedings with what looked like amusement. When he leaned in to say hello, the air crackled.

I dropped the leash. Mistress Cherry slinked off somewhere into the night. I may still have been strapped into her clothes, but I didn't need her crowding in and getting in between Douglas and me. When Cherry smiled, she bared her teeth like a predator—come in, but not too close. She sat poised and arch, inside an invisible cage out of which she could swipe a claw and never be touched back. Everything in *my* body softened, slumped toward him, and grinned like a toddler. Cartoon butterflies may have in fact flapped out of my ears, nose, and mouth. Forty-five minutes later, I definitely kissed him first, but he kissed me right back. Midway through the next morning, there was even an e-mail:

> Kat of the crop and pony-hair boots, SO GREAT to meet
> you in person. I can't say exactly what it is—there is this very
> palpable spark! . . . See you tonight.

Not just me, then.

And still, my brain spat nastiness at me on the way to the wine bar to meet him. You're just blinded by your neediness, you stupid girl. He can't be as handsome as you thought he was in the half-light of that club. You hadn't been kissed for months, so anything would seem good to you. Sure, he says he has friends, and your creepy Google stalking seems to indicate that he's actually got the job he says he does, but if that's really true, why would he bother with the likes of you? Have a drink, maybe make out a little, keep your distance. Mistress Cherry concurred. Fine—have your fun, but don't expect me to pity you when he smashes you to a pulp. You know it's coming and I'm just trying to warn you. Besides, he probably won't even show up.

I stood on the sidewalk outside for a moment, inhaled, and set my jaw. He was already inside, and even impossibly cuter than he'd been the night before—now stripped of the hard leather shell and swaddled in a gray, fuzzy sweater with a goofily grinning skull knitted into it. Do sociopaths own novelty winter wear? I wondered. I followed him downstairs to a basement couch. We ordered drinks. He cleared his throat. "I have something I want to get out of the way . . ."

While Effexor is halfway decent at blunting the immediate physical reactions to panic, I felt them like phantom pains. Of course there's something to get out of the way. Of course. My body hunched forward to block the blow of whatever was coming next. Cherry snapped it back into place, rigid spine and a frozen smile. "Oh?"

"I just wanted to be up front that I was married before, got divorced about ten years ago when I was twenty-eight, and then was engaged again, and that ended pretty compassionately. I took a year off from dating so I could work on myself and, well, here we are." He paused, waiting to see how that landed.

"Any . . . kids?"

"Nope."

"Want any?"

"Not really. You?"

I exhaled and curled my right pinkie around his left. "Never wanted them and I don't think that will ever change."

He seemed relieved, not disgusted or bored by my presence so far as I could tell. Our drinks arrived. Cheers, big swallow. "And I suppose I should return the favor and be straight with you . . ."

"Oh?"

"I don't know quite how to explain this, but I have some . . . issues. Some of them just because I have them, and I swear I see a shrink and I am on meds, but some got a lot worse a little while back."

"Tell me."

And I did—the version I'd rehearsed and recited so many times in an attempt to explain to people why I didn't really want to date, why I flinched, got sad, and left parties early if I went at all. That I had issues with anxiety and depression. And that I was lied to by someone I thought I loved—starting with his name—and the next person I tried to date did the same thing. I braced myself for the look of pity. He pulled out his wallet—date over, I guess.

He handed me his license. "See, my name is really Douglas. If you want, I will write down my sister's name and number and my best friend's if you'd like. He's a lawyer. You can call them. I want you to know you can trust me."

I didn't take him up on the offer, but I was awfully grateful that he'd made it. He saw me for the flinching, tender soul I was behind my high, hard boots and bloodred lipstick and he wanted to let me know that he liked me despite it—and because of it. Hell, he just liked ME and he didn't mind that I knew it. That sure felt like a first.

Falling in love with Douglas is the easiest thing I have ever done. The moment he opened his mouth and whispered into my ear, all the twitching, whizzing, fretting atoms in my body shifted over just a little bit, slipped into place, and, at last, relaxed. I felt gleeful and graceful and settled in my skin for the first time I could remember, tuned into the unfamiliar and wholly welcome bliss of someone whose soul buzzed on the same frequency as mine. He felt it, too—I knew it because he told me. He TOLD me, said the words out loud so I could hear them loud and clear, etch them onto my bones, and run my fingers over them. God, I felt loved and I gave as good as I got.

I'd been the first one to say "I love you." I couldn't hold it in any longer. For weeks, the phrase had been thrumming in my thoughts so constantly I was surprised it hadn't manifested in three-inch letters across my forehead. Still, I had paid the price for saying them before—and to people who deserved them far less.

It costs something to say it for the first time, mostly because you're taking a risk on the exchange rate. Those three words don't hold the same worth for everyone. Some hesitate to spend them— either holding them in reserve so as not to devalue, staving off buyer's remorse, or just not having much extra to spare. Some people are careless. Some people lie. Some people just suck.

I'd seen no evidence of any of those characteristics, but then again, I'd not exactly proven myself to be a reliable judge of late. I dammed the words back, waiting for proof that the man in my head was the one who actually walked the earth. The proof came in the form of his friends—a tight knot of them who he'd known since his early twenties, and who clearly adored him.

Douglas and I hosted a party at his apartment. While I poured flaming blue cocktails and he guarded fancy cheese from his whippet and Irish wolfhound's jaws, I watched them watch him watching me. I knew then it was safe to let go.

Later that night in the calm dark of his bedroom, "I love you" kicked its way past my heart, my throat, my tongue, and my teeth. My words hung in the air for only a fraction of a second before they crashed into his, echoing the same thing. His feelings were mine, for me, and I wanted to be brave enough to believe them.

Even if someone is easy to love, that doesn't necessarily take the gravity and terror out of the situation. Toss yourself out of an airplane and the most natural thing to do is fall. It's not as if resisting is going to get you anywhere.

And we both braced for impact, all the time. I could see it in the little pauses before our carefully selected words, the flinch before each revelation of a flaw, the almost overeager need to please and serve—as if our presence wasn't present enough. Is that okay with you? Do you need anything? Do you mind if I . . . ? What can I get for you?

Is that enough? Am I enough? I'm terrified that you'll stop loving me. Please don't.

We'd both grown up as weird kids in places we didn't belong. In his case, it was as a New Wave kid in a preppy Southern town where boys who favored theater and dancing over sports were looked at as somewhat suspect—if not flat-out tortured. Having a much older dad who drank his share of Scotch and then some, and a too-young marriage to a woman who favored the same made him feel tolerated more than loved, and barely even that. A broken engagement after that left him even more unsure of his value outside of a steady paycheck, and I could tell he worried constantly about being too conventional and routine-oriented for me. I made it my mission to calm him, and let him know he wasn't just plenty—he was far more than I'd ever had. And to my utter shock, he did the same.

I almost didn't recognize myself in this skin—smiling all the time, guts at rest, and mind at ease. The battery-acid stomach I'd lived with was somehow neutralized. How could this possibly be love if I wasn't constantly worried that Douglas was going away? That I would finally let my guard down, show my raw, weird, wounded, worried self, and he'd recoil in horror or fade away.

He just . . . didn't. Not when I told him I saw a therapist every week. Not when I told him I took medication to keep my brain from screaming. Not when I had the flu. Not when I cried. Not when I flinched in the passenger's seat. Not when I told him about my mother.

Still, one more layer to peel back.

After six months, my parents wanted to meet him. They hadn't met every man I'd dated for a significant time, and none of them more than once. Usually at a graduation. Steven, whom I'd been with longer than anyone, had nearly ducked out on meeting Pup when he'd come to town for a business meeting ("I don't *do* family."), but was shamed into it at the last minute by our mutual friends who were coming along with or without him. While Douglas had no such qualms, I wasn't exactly champing at the bit for this part of the puzzle to be placed.

It's one thing to describe your mother's unwellness, choosing words to cushion the broken edges so they scrape a little less coming out and sinking in. It's another for the people to see it in full flower, emanating from a face that foretells your future. Not that I truly believed they'd actually go through with the trip. Dates were set and tickets were bought—to the airport nearest Douglas's place upstate, not Brooklyn, because the bustle was deemed too much—but I didn't believe my parents would actually manifest. But sure enough, word spread around the little town after Pup booked the handicapped-accessible suite at the small hotel in the center of town.

"Sooooo, meeting the parents, huh? Big step for you two lovebirds."

"What are you crazy kids going to do while they're here? Some sightseeing? Maybe Cooperstown? Just walking around town?"

I did my best to staple a smile on my cheeks. "Mmm-hmm. If they actually make it here."

"Why would you think they wouldn't? Of course they want to see you and meet Douglas!"

I can want a unicorn that vomits Susan B. Anthony dollars, but that doesn't mean I'm going to find one tapping on my front window with her horn. Something inside me just couldn't ration that quantity of hope. And good thing, too.

A day or two before their arrival, Pup sent an e-mail, worded as gently as he could. The anxiety over the travel, the unfamiliar town, her sinful daughter's sinful life (I assumed that last part)—it pinned her to the bed and left her unfit for flight. I clenched my jaw, lifted up the corner of my mouth in a rueful grin, typed back a measured "That's okay . . . whenever she's better" and told Douglas he could stop loving me now if he needed to. You've seen what's in store. Get out while you can.

He held me until I stopped shaking.

Two weeks later, at the arrivals gate at Albany International Airport, Mumsie looked like a paper doll, traced over on onionskin and nestled into the wheelchair Pup pushed gently down the hallway. I'd nearly pulled Douglas's Jeep over to the shoulder of the highway at least three times on my way to pick them up, hyperventilating and terrified of weaving into highway traffic. I was ashamed of myself for being terrified to see her, unsure of which version we would receive: the shrieking knot of need and pain and accusation, the pharmaceutically sogged corpse melted into the couch, or most chest-wrenching of all, the marionette, slumped in her chair, occasionally flickering to life in an eerie approximation of the mother I missed so fiercely, then dimming, slackening just as quickly.

It was the last one who came to visit that time. And I could tell she was trying—or at least that's what I told myself. That she was using all she had left to capture a snapshot of what her daughter's life was and would be with this man.

Douglas was gentle with her, and I loved him even more for it. Both because I gave a damn about her comfort, and because it felt like his embrace of my inevitable. This is the ghost of future present, O boyfriend mine. Boo! Have we scared you off? How about now when we lumber, sloth slow, across the dining room and need the menu read to us? Or when we take half a minute to answer a yes/no question, take a second afternoon nap to recover from all the sitting around, and startle at the sound of the neighbor's lawn mower. Still here? Why? You're allowed to leave.

Pup, as their spokesperson, spoke in the plural afterward. We loved meeting Douglas. We think those dogs are so elegant (and Douglas should really add a railing to those stairs so no one falls off in the dark). We think the two of you are such a great match.

I did, too. I really did. And I was fine with whatever I was allotted, heartwise. I felt so greedy, what with the "knowing my boyfriend's real name" and the "I love yous" and the seeing him more than a couple of hours a week without being made to feel like I was sapping his precious solitude. I couldn't possibly ask for more. I didn't need much more. But was that really true?

In my life before this, I wasn't especially keen to share relationship worries with many people for fear that my paranoiac theories and doubts would be confirmed, but this time, I was taking no chances. I sought advice from a few friends and my therapist about the best way to ask for a State of the Union address without scaring Douglas off. "It's okay," I assured them/me. "It is A-OHHHKAAAAYYYY if he never wants to marry me. I am fine with things just the way they are." While I supported the institution wholeheartedly (plus, yay, cake), happily-ever-after in a marshmallow dress just didn't actually apply to me. That was for the lovable, clean-fingernailed girls who managed to slither into run-free tights most mornings, melted at the sight of infants, and didn't have brimstone-breathed demons in their brains whispering their every fault to them each waking hour.

But I had to know—just be certain how much hope for the future I was allowed to have. I could tuck the rest in a box and dole it out to friends. What I had was more than I'd ever had before: more love, more care, more safety. I would be fine with or without marriage and I would stay so very happily for as long as he'd have me. But the worry that he wouldn't have me was starting to eat me alive.

Just ask him, my friends and the good doctor said. This is the happiest we've ever seen you, and we suspect you'll like the answer. But are you prepared for what happens if it's not the one you want?

Prepared? HA! That's all I do is prepare. That's what I'm built for. I spend all of my waking moments (and a good chunk of sleeping ones, too) putting hammer, nails, scratched skin, and blood into constructing the worst-case scenario and armoring for battle against it.

Not just the big stuff—love and work and real estate—but everything from the route between the subway door and me to scoring a decent seat at the movies to finding the party host to say good night to how late to work I'd be if I hit the snooze alarm another time.

I needed to know. So after a few fretful weeks and a substantial amount of wine, I found my moment, standing a dozen feet or so away in the kitchen of the church he'd bought in upstate New York and was turning into a weekend home, my arms crossed around my rib cage, eyes anywhere but on his. "Sooooo . . . do you think you'd ever get married again?"

Douglas doesn't always answer questions the second he's asked. It's a thing I quickly became used to, but right then, every millisecond he breathed in pressed the air out of me in little bursts, snapping like Bubble Wrap, asphyxiating my hope.

He spoke. "Probably."

And then he disappeared. Not right that second, but in a slow fade over the next couple of weeks, manifesting mostly in missed calls and "Sorry, I'm still stuck at the office" and couch naps and early bedtimes. Though several of my life decisions were close contenders, asking for more from my boyfriend had clearly been the most laughable to the universe. Why couldn't I just have held my tongue and been content? Could I take that moment back? Make a show of cool-girl insouciance, let him know that, hey man, we're good here? Whatevs.

But I was me. So on the year-and-a-half anniversary of our first date, as I sat wet-haired on our battered tapestry couch, and he lowered himself next to me and started apologizing, I was almost proud of myself for not being blindsided. Here comes the secret wife (can lightning strike twice?), the work affair, the boundary of his love that I've run up against. It's okay; it was sublime while it lasted. Thank you for letting me love you for a little while.

But that's not what he was saying. Not the text, not the subtext, not at all.

"I'm so sorry," he was saying, "for being so wrapped up in work and not present enough for you or as much as I want to be. I love our life together. Will you marry me?"

There was a box. And a ring. And the demon hissing in my ear, "He feels sorry for you because you made such a fool of yourself, asking about marriage that night. He's just letting you save face. Why would a good man saddle himself with the likes of you?"

"You don't . . . have to . . ." I stuttered.

He stared at me, confused. "What are you talking about?"

And all at once I saw it: he needed me as much as I needed him.

"I mean, yes. Thank you. Yes, please."

And as he slipped the ring onto my finger—a placeholder for now, just something he thought I would like until I picked out my own because I'd be wearing it for the rest of eternity—my head slowly detached from my body, floating a few feet up and away, smiling down to see what I looked like when I'm at peace.

IRRATIONAL FEAR #5
GETTING MY HAIR CUT

My hair goes down to my waist and I trim my bangs myself. Very few people know how long it is because it's almost inevitably up in a bun. It's my signature look at this point, and has been since I wore it live on CNN one Fourth of July while talking about competitive eating. People took notice, and I do actually like it. It's also my anxiety, hiding in plain sight, high atop my head as a statement of personal style.

I can't stand to get my hair cut. It's not the loss of length (I've shaved it almost down to the skull with a Bic razor, burned most of it off in a pathetic home-bleaching incident the night before a first date, and can lop seven inches onto the bathroom floor with minimal trauma) or the fear of a rotten cut. (I've weathered plenty of those: see me ages two to eighteen. It grows back.) It's that all the moving parts that make up a salon visit cause me to grab the scissors myself.

Booking the appointment: it's been made easier by the Internet, but this action sets the clock ticking. If the appointment is on a weekend, that means that I have to be at a certain place at a certain time, and all the hours before it are effectively useless. I can't start writing, working, relaxing, reading a book, cooking a meal, or doing much but muck around on social media until it's time to leave my house. Sure, I could schedule the cut for first thing in the morning, but then I'd be unable to sleep, worried that I'll miss the alarm. If the appointment is during the week, I'm terrified I won't be able to tie up loose ends before I would need to leave work. And then work will be mad and I'll get fired and then I'll just have to sell my hair for cash anyhow.

I'm not exactly sure what I think is going to happen if I stroll into the salon a little late. Yes, it's disrespectful and has a domino effect on the stylist's other clients, but do I think I'm going to be berated? Shamed? Stabbed with pinking shears? That's never happened to me before, but there's always a first time. Plus, Sweeney Todd.

Chatting: I fear being insufficiently delightful when speaking to the stylist—especially with someone who holds my visual fate in their hands. If I cannot sparkle and charm, will I be issued the dreaded Dorothy Hamill 'do that haunted my youth? I fear that if I point to a Dita Von Teese or Bettie Page, I'll hear an intake of breath through the teeth, "Oh, honey, no. Not with your [an up-and-down scan] everything."

Pop culture paints modern womanhood as a decoupage of manis, pedis, blowouts, spa treatments, and other aesthetic services lacquered onto one's person by a gaggle of "Oh, gurrrrlll!" divas, but that's never flown with me. It's reductive and unkind to make someone into your Greek chorus, your flock of Cinderella-dressing bluebirds. There's a person standing with their torso just inches from your eyes. It's intimate, so treat them like a human being—even if you're not feeling like much of a person that day. And if I'm not, it feels deeply awkward to go to the salon at all.

Pampering in general: I've always admired the moxie of the

"because I'm worth it" crowd, but I don't always buy it for myself. Literally: I can't bring myself to buy a service that benefits only me. It might be a lapsed-Catholic thing, ground into my skin by ascetic nuns who used the same bar of soap for their body, face, hair, and possibly dishes, but spending cash on spas, massages, nails, and schmancy haircuts just feels to me like tempting fate. "Oh, look at yoooouuuuu, vain girl, thinking you've got a shot in hell of looking like a grown-up adult human lady person. Yeah, go ahead and spend that money on nail polish you'll just chip, on bangs that will grow out, muscles that will kink on the subway ride home. You might feel pretty for just a second, but you're the same ugly, awkward girl you always were. Why waste? Why bother?"

Tipping: I've lived in New York since 1996 and had been going to restaurants, bars, coffee shops, and salons since one thousand years before that. I live in horror of under-tipping, and it's almost a religion in this town. In food or drink situations, it's pretty straight-forward, you add it to the check or jar and you go on your well-fed way. In a salon, there are multiple handlers of your head, enve-lopes, owners—wait, did I bring cash? Did I leave enough? Did I undertip and seem cheap so that next time I come I'll get lousy ser-vice? Did I overtip and look like a rube who doesn't know the rules? If I screwed that up either way, I can never show my face here again.

Best to reach for the scissors and cut out the middleman.

CHAPTER EIGHT

Drugging the Beast

There are twelve low-dose generic Xanax pills rattling around in a pill bottle in my purse. Just a few millimeters of plastic and my quivering hands stand between a full-skin hurricane and tranquil seas, and I can very rarely bring myself to break the seal and swim to safety.

It took me seven and a half years to make the appointment, ten days to walk into the pharmacy with the prescription, thirty minutes to fretfully stroll the aisles and debate the appeal of various nail-polish colors and formulas before sliding it across the counter, three days to collect it (despite the pharmacist's blithe assurance that I could just stick around for twenty minutes), and a solid month and a half to deem a situation dire enough to say "uncle."

I was too far gone for the tiny pill to do any good. I'd lain in bed half the night with a pulse so jangled, breath so strangled I could feel the panic in my eyeballs, fingertips, the soles of my feet, while Douglas breathed rhythmically next to me, oblivious. I had no good reason, it was just something for my jackrabbit brain to do. I crept down the stairs to where my purse was hanging on a hook near the front door, fumbled at the twist cap in the dark, feeling as if I'd failed someone. If the pill tamped down my pulse, unknotted my muscles, or muffled the clangor of my awful thoughts, I didn't notice.

If it had, no one else in the world would begrudge me the relief—okay, maybe some antipharma activists or Tom Cruise or religious zealots who damn drugs they don't understand because they've never had cause to. But they don't have to live in my body. Lucky them.

As previously mentioned, I was fourteen the first time I was given pills to manage my moods. I had fallen prey to a bout of severe depression and was carted away to sessions with a silken-voiced psychiatrist who doled out some fairly empathetic counseling from the depths of her squishy leather chair—alongside some tricyclic antidepressants she assured me would lend a "gentle lift" to my emotional state.

And they almost did, right over the railing of a third-floor staircase at the high school to which I soon made a reluctant return. It was fine. Whatever. I guess we're doing this. But it didn't take a doctoral degree to link the doorstopper-sized pills to the constipation that bricked my bowels to the point of agony, the leaching of all moisture from my tongue (to this day, I can still identify a meds-induced mouth click from halfway across the room), and the bouts of vertigo that struck at highly inconvenient times and locales. Like, say, the landing outside Intro to Biology just as third period was letting out. I steered myself out of the flow of navy-skirted and dress-slacked bodies and anchored the bottom of my rib cage against the metal railing. When you're that dizzy, down seems just as good as up. I flushed the rest of the bottle (and almost the bottle, itself) that day and no one ever bothered me about them again.

But . . . BUT! Just because you're off meds doesn't mean you've got it all solved, that you've bested the beast through the sheer force of your will. For millions of people who want and ought to take them, it's a sickening merry-go-round of economic denial. The very conditions they treat can make it difficult to get or hold the jobs that might provide the insurance that would cover both the care and the medications themselves. If you're feeling too wretched to get out of bed, too panicked to breach the doorway to physically get there (or boot up the computer to log on to your e-mail), and unable to concentrate once you have, it's damned difficult to have any sort of job security. And even if you do have the luxury of a regular wage, that's not an assurance of quality care, or that your insurance company will cover your particular prescription without an astronomic copay. Or that your family, colleagues, and community will approve or understand.

And sometimes, the drugs just don't work for you.

When I was thirty years old, I went through the breakup that threatened to end me. After several months of waking up nauseated and screaming, I went to my physician, who seemed to take my acquiescence on the meds front as a personal victory. I talk fast. I'm animated. Sometimes agitated when I'm in a doctor's office because it's a particular trigger point for me (see: years of Mumsie-related waiting room hours, logged)—and over the years I'd been her patient, she'd taken it on as a cause.

As the steward of my gynecological health as well, she had a pretty rational reason to be invested in the state of my dating life, but had the tendency to take things a bit too far for my comfort. "So you're seeing a new guy, huh? How does he . . . deal with all your energy? Should we get you something to take you down a notch?" "Dating again? Are you sure you don't want something to make you a little . . . easier to be around? Don't want to scare anyone off!" (The me of today would have kicked her to the curb and considered writing a truly scathing online review to make sure that no one else would weather her judgmental bedside manner. Me then—nodded and agreed.) So when I came in seeking something, anything, that would short-circuit the morning (and afternoon and evening) horror cycle, she practically threw sparks, wringing her hands with glee. We (she) arrived at Effexor XR, a long-release SNRI that so far as she knew had no nasty side effects, like the vertigo, constipation, and dry mouth, or the sexual dampening, mental muddiness, and weight gain others I'd known had faced on mood-altering drugs.

I just want to still be ME, you know? I told her. Just without the daily screaming sadness, acid stomach, and leaden despair if at all possible.

Lift and lightening, she promised. The edges blunted. Maybe a bit less electric chattiness from me, but that's what we want, yes? Yes, I suppose we do, because look where that got me. Thank you.

While the medicine did jack squat for my bouts of depression, for the first time in my life, my first reaction to every small conflict—real or imagined—wasn't a blazing stomachache and the immediate impulse to apologize and find fault in myself.

Unless a person has spent some portion of their existence dragged around by a fist knotted through their intestines, they may not grasp the euphoria of that development. It is a wretched thing to be a slave to your body's chemistry. It lies to you, stoking fear and guilt and horror where none is called for, turning shadows to predators and neutral interactions into mental films played on endless loop so you can dissect the moment that you screwed everything up forever. Having a magic pill tamp down the acid and tremor before they start to cycle—maybe even stop them from firing up their engines in the first place? Unthinkable, and thank you, thank you, thank you, modern science. For as long as it lasts.

For the first while, I touted its benefits to anyone who would listen. Probably annoyingly often, but I didn't much care. It HURTS, being anxious. The stomach roiling, jaw clenching, cheek biting, finger picking, muscle tensing, and headaches take their toll, and my impulse had always been to do whatever I could to make it stop as swiftly as possible. Assume guilt, apologize, rectify, appease, even if it came at a cost. Mumsie's crying? I'm so sorry, what did I do? Boyfriend seems distant? It can't be because he's stressed about work, it must be because I've been too needy—or possibly fundamentally unlovable. I'll work on that. Someone else got the assignment I wanted? I suck, I suck, I suck. Must work through the night and not sleep. Ever.

With the physical symptoms subdued, I was newly able to see my place in the world, and shockingly enough, it wasn't always as the bumbler, screw-up, term-limited-lovable, messy kid I'd come to believe I was. Perhaps . . . perhaps I'd let some people into my life who had a vested interest in making me believe those things. But no more.

The thing about these meds is that sometimes they just stop working. They can be life-changing, life-SAVING for people, pull them back from the abyss, and make them themselves again, or in my case, give me a self I'd never known I could be. And then they flicker out. Morph. Get greedy for more brain space. The side effects had, thank God, been relatively mild—an acceptable exchange for the relief from the nervous cycling that had defined just about every facet of my life.

The "zaps," for instance. Picture a chilly November night in your childhood. You're nestled in a bed heaped with fuzzy blankets and pull the top one up to rearrange it. In the dark, it throws flashes—a field full of fireflies, only you can feel a sharp little shock.

Now imagine that happening inside your skull, without warning, as you're walking down the street. The first time it happens, you think you're going insane. That never quite wears off, but at least you know what you're in for. Effexor XR (which can be prescribed generically as venlafaxine hydrochloride) has what's called a short half-life, meaning that the rate at which it's absorbed into the body is slower than the rate at which it's eliminated. The way that plays out is that if after taking 150 milligrams per days for a few years you miss your dosage schedule by even a little bit—forty-five minutes, for some of us—the neurotransmitters in your brain, especially the ones involving serotonin, alter the way they're conducting energy. And you can feel it.

Like when you're headed to dinner in Las Vegas with your friend and her parents and it's in a different time zone than the one you usually live in and you have to rush back to your hotel room and gobble a pill when you suddenly realize that the bright, strobing lights weren't actually part of the Strip's bombast. (The call is coming from insiiiide your heeeaaaaaad . . .) Or when you stayed over at your boyfriend's house without planning properly and find yourself on the subway home at 3 A.M., hoping you won't miss your stop because you were too distracted by the flashbulbs popping in your head. Or when you sit for hours upon hours in a British National Health clinic, sickened and ashamed that you miscounted the number of pills to bring with you, and the only balm for your brain is sitting on your bathroom sink 3,500 miles away, across an ocean. Or when you're sobbing to the callow, impassive pharmacist's assistant that pleasepleaseplease you need her to try your doctor's number again because things will get very, very bad for you if you run out tomorrow. ("I don't have time to deal with this right now," she will tell you, and you will feel more like a crazy person than you have ever felt in your life. And you will sob even harder when you ask for her supervisor and he tells you he does have time for you and these pills will tide you over and this seems like the kindest gift anyone has ever bestowed upon your sorry, insane self.)

That was tolerable-ish, especially since I could easily pin blame on my own carelessness—a habit I'd been perfecting since birth. I could also self-lash over the fact that my clothes didn't fit anymore. That I felt bloated and lumpen despite not having changed my eating habits in any appreciable way, and that only the nearly complete elimination of food and extraordinary amounts of exercise made any sort of reduction in my mass. I stopped looking in mirrors and ducked cameras, walked hunched past reflective surfaces to avoid looking at the smeared version of myself I'd become. I could have lived with that—an unpleasant, but somewhat acceptable price to pay for delivery from the constant, physical agony of anxiety—but then the drug started to shirk that end of the bargain, too.

Effexor XR had never done much to lift me from the dank depths of depression and now the fret and pick and sting of worry were starting to creep back in. So far as my physician was concerned, that simply meant more of the drug was required. I wasn't convinced. I knew the cost.

When I talk about Mumsie, I'll say she's unwell. That's all anyone really needs to know, and generally all I will offer, but people often want more—a specific diagnosis. I think it mostly comes from a good place, rather than just morbid curiosity (though there's been plenty of that, too). If you give something a name, they know where to start the conversation. "Oh, my cousin had that." "I had a teacher who went through that." "I went through that and here's what helped—or didn't." For her, there's no single diagnosis, and even if there were, it's not really mine to share and she's not especially askable anymore.

And if there were, she'd also be treatable. Doctors wouldn't have, long ago, begun burying her body and brain under layers of medication so thick that it's usually hard to see if she's still in there. Some of the drugs are to quell the physical pain that she's lived with as long as I have been aware. But the rest of the drugs? Where do I begin?

As lashing as her rages could be, I knew them and could still find my mother at the center of the maelstrom. When I came home that first winter break from college after she'd been hospitalized, I couldn't find her anymore and I flailed, trying. Her body was there on the couch pretty constantly in the daylight hours. Some part of her muscle memory noted the fact that her daughters were home for the holidays and wanted to be present for the festivities (such as they were that year), but the drugs wouldn't let her stay awake. Or alive in a way I understood. I reached into the swirling fog, tried to twine on to the gossamer strands of the mother I knew, and they'd simply blow through my fingers. After a while, I had to stop reaching. It just hurt too much.

Twenty-five years later, the drugs are her, and she they. Whatever thread snapped loose that autumn that I left home was knitted into the prescriptions that wind around her, bandaging her in place. I have seen what happens when they are pried loose, and it is cruel.

One of them is (or was) Effexor XR. Once when she was taken off it—and all her other medications—following a medical procedure some years back, I went to see her in a hospital ER and she did not know me. I am not sure she knew her own name, the town, the city, the country, the galaxy she was in, just that the nurses were trying to poison her with stew and leathery green beans (to be fair, from the way they looked and smelled, that was not an unfair assessment). She was tied to the bed. Another time, in the meds purge after another sickness, she stared straight through me, craning to see the train she expected to come steaming through the center of her room in the geriatric psych ward. She alternated between fretting that she didn't have enough money for the fare, and horror that it would not slow, would just crush her in its path. I wanted to save her. She could not see me. It was the worst I had ever felt.

Until.

It was time for me to get off the Effexor Express. I just couldn't let it have me anymore, risk buying a ticket on that same trip, but I'd seen what had happened when people tried to disembark. One friend who'd lost his insurance along with his job found himself in no state to negotiate a plan with his caregivers, so he went off it cold turkey. By the end of the third day, he was afraid to leave his bedroom for fear of finding that he had, in fact, not hallucinated plunging a butcher's knife into his infant daughter's innocent belly. Another told me she'd hunkered, starving and sick, in her apartment for nearly a month after taking her last pill. The vertigo that pinned her to the bed was the only force that kept her from stumbling into the kitchen for a sharp enough object to make it all stop. So perhaps a different route was required.

But I didn't trust my doctor to provide the proper road map. I've found out in the eight years since then that a physician "breakup" is not an uncommon side effect of quitting Effexor. Perhaps it's baby/bathwater irrationality exercised by a patient with a temporarily short-circuiting brain, but I just couldn't face her for fear I'd shake her, scream, and fall under her spell. She's a doctor. She knows best, yes? And if not, why have I been allowing her to pour poison on my brain? Better go it alone . . . or online.

I steered down every electronic byway and message board, seeking flares sent up by people who had made it to the other side safely(ish).

Few, it seemed, emerged wholly unscarred, and those who did had mainly arrived there via a method they called the Bridge: slowly transitioning from Effexor XR use to Prozac. I was pleased they'd made their safe passage, but seeing as how Prozac wasn't then and isn't yet available on drugstore shelves or in my grocer's freezer, I couldn't consider it as an option. Or stepping down to lower and lower doses, because that would require a new prescription and I would have to go to my doctor. So, I dove off the cliff with my Internet crash helmet on a Sunday evening in early July 2007, when I began my tapering-off plan, which I estimated would take ten weeks, dropping my dosage by 10 percent each week. Seems reasonable enough, right? Surely it was less precipitous a drop than the 25 percent most doctors (per my diligent, secondhand research indicated) would advise. I'd planned to keep detailed notes throughout the whole process, documenting changes in mood, sex drive, crying, sleep, exercise, and other indicators of wellness and sharing them on an anonymous blog in case anyone cared to follow along—or possibly pull me back to shore.

SUNDAY, JULY 8, 2007

DAY 1

Sex: Yes

Tears: Yes (of happiness, though—the sex was good, and I met my pals' brand-new baby).

Booze: 1 martini

Sleep: woken by the larger dog at 7-ish A.M. No naps.

Exercise: 35 min. Dog Walk / Installed A/C

Mood: Variable. (Good movie, good company, good dinner, good sex, bad PMS)

Effexor Dose: OJ Method (.9 glass of 10-oz. OJ w/ 150mg Effexor XR = approx 135 mg)

The "OJ Method," which I'd seen vouched for on several message boards, involved opening a capsule, pouring all of the beads into a glass of orange juice, and drinking nine-tenths of it for the first week, eight-tenths the next, and so on. Easy peasy, fresh-juice squeezy—just sip my ever-decreasing fill each night, and in two and a half months, a bright, shiny, reclaimed brain awaited me on the horizon.

This was the next entry:

TUESDAY, SEPTEMBER 18, 2007

DAY 70

Took my final dose (10 mg) this past Saturday, and today, I feel as if I'm not in physical control of much of anything above my shoulders. My mind is clear-ish, but my brain is being violently shocked, and I'm dizzy, nauseated, twitchy, and in a great deal of pain from a stabbing headache. Would very much like to go out to find something to eat, but I'm having a great deal of difficulty standing up and walking in a straight line.

When all of this is finally exorcised from my body, I will make it my sworn mission to let people—friends, strangers who stumble across this account on the Internet, anyone who needs to—know that they should never even contemplate starting to take Effexor XR, because no matter any benefits it may have, the withdrawal is too large a price to pay.

Day 70: Addendum

"When people suddenly stop using EFFEXOR XR, they can get symptoms from stopping the medicine too fast."

Seeing as it's, well, DAY 70 of my tapering off and I'm

having such violent reactions, I'm going to make a bold
statement and say that there is NO SUCH THING as
slow enough. The "too fast" in the Wyeth statement above
slyly places the blame on the consumer, rather than the
manufacturer. Jerks.

I cut out the juice pretty quickly, both reeling from the sugar
spike and frightened of an imprecise dose. The first few weeks went
rather uneventfully—a twitch here, a dizzy spell there.

And then I lost my mind. Or maybe my body. It was impossible
to tell in the thick of it, in a meeting in my new boss's office having to squash my eyelids shut and cling to the chair while a vertigo
attack turned the room into a theme-park rotor ride. (That was a
fun conversation: "Um, I know I just started here and thank you for
hiring me and I think I'll actually probably be good at this but right
now I am going through psychiatric drug withdrawal and trying not
to barf on your carpet.")

In a fire throat scream to Douglas to pull over the Jeep on the New
York State Thruway because I needed to dry-heave on the pebble-
strewn shoulder. In the nightmares where every perceived screw-up
and social gaffe I'd made since birth was in surround sound and a
Technicolor broadcast in my brain and catastrophized the second I
attempted sleep each night. In the two-minute, pedestrian-choked
walk between the Rockefeller Center subway stop and my office
door where every blink, step, gesture felt like a flash bomb detonat-
ing in my face. In the stomach-sick, rot-brain, dizzy-headed, sweat-
soaked-sheet hours when I was sure the kindest thing I could do for
myself and humanity was to remove myself from it. But couldn't
get up from bed to walk to the bathroom to get the pills, scissors, or
blades.

And oh god oh god oh god, poor Douglas, who had to deal with me. I told few people, I was so ashamed—and just drifted from contact with anyone else who loved me. Somehow I managed to move my bones and muscles to work because I needed to prove my worth to the world in some way. Imagine your brain as a raw pork shoulder (or a steamed head of cauliflower, if that's your bag) in a round glass fishbowl. Now spin it, and then grab the sides to slow it. (Just go with it. It made sense at the time.) The inside keeps rotating. That's what it felt like to move, so I didn't.

Not that it was much more pleasant to lie there, desiccating from the inside, knowing that I'd never be sane again. In the end, it took nine months to feel anywhere close to healthy again, two years for the final zap to strike, and never for the anger to abate.

I know and love plenty of people for whom various prescription medications have been a godsend. It's given them back their lives, relationships, brains, and bodies. I root for them loudly, avidly, and envy them, but I just can't bring myself to join their ranks. Not full-time at least. I know that seems silly, or at least self-sabotaging. Everyone's on something, right? Or maybe it just seems that way to me because friends and strangers alike have no qualms about sidling up at a party or slipping into my Twitter or Facebook messages to tell me about the new drug they've been prescribed, and how it has made them able to function again, or even for the first time ever. I felt that way about Effexor for the first few years before it backfired on me, and it gave rise to a few brand-new phobias for me: a fear that the meds won't work, that the side effects will be untenable, or that they'll work too well and I won't be able to quit.

Cymbalta and Pristiq are in the same SNRI gang as Effexor, so their name is effectively mud to me (though I'm sure they have their fans). I hear excellent things about SSRIs like Lexapro, Prozac, Celexa, and Zoloft, that they offer light and lift, but their sister medication, Paxil, has been known to bring on those damnable zaps, so they're off the menu for me, too. (I never claimed this was rational.) BuSpar seems chill as heck, but seems to come with a fair amount of side effects. And benzos—like Valium, Klonopin, Xanax, and Ativan—they work well. So well. Too well for a lot of people (some of whom I love very much), who then struggle painfully to kick them. I fear becoming one of them.

In the less-than-three months between my engagement and wedding, I gritted my teeth and accepted a prescription for Ativan to be taken as needed to take the edge off my anxiety. (The need was apparently so great that an acquaintance I ran into on the subway refused to leave my side or let me onto the train until I downed one in front of her.) It took over a year for me to finish off the bottle, then nearly another eight years to contemplate any sort of chemical intervention on my own behalf. This is not rational, but knowing that does not help, just flings me further toward the center of the spiral. You can't even take basic care of yourself? What a burden you are. What a pitiful soul.

I finally gave in and saw a doctor because I was not well. Not in an acute, life-ending way, but a slow leak. And not for me, mind you—my comfort alone would not be reason enough, but because I knew it harmed Douglas to watch me be so cruel to myself—staying awake for days if I thought I hadn't earned my keep in the world, hunched over with tensed, twitching muscles, afraid of being caught off guard and unprepared for something that was needed from me, picking at my thumbs until blood stained my hands.

So, I went to see an empathetic RN I started thinking of as the Witch Doctor. (In a totally nice way.)

"Leaky gut!" she said, and I nodded enthusiastically. (She

wore striped tights, had pointy glasses, and called me Kitten, and I respond very well to that when I'm afraid.) "Saliva tests!" (Yes, YES! It's fun to spit—much more so than bleeding.) "I'm going to take so much blood from you!" (Okay, if you must.) "Elimination diet!" (Hrrrrmmm.)

"What if you're not really anxious? What if it's been your thyroid or a vitamin deficiency this whole time?" Yes, what if?

She linked arms with me and skipped to the front desk to settle my bill and collect my paperwork. I felt like a jerk. Not because of the skipping (that was pretty delightful), but let's say I had been misreading my own brain and body this whole time and simply suffering because I'd been too scared to act on my own behalf. She eased me off the hook there, too, and this was the magic of the Witch Doctor. "You have gotten bad care. My heart aches for you. I want to change that. With you."

Deep breath: okay.

I left her office hopeful and confused. If I wasn't actually anxious—not in the way I'd understood for so much of my life— then what was I? Who was I? You get a notion of yourself, for good or for bad, and everything forms around that. This trembling core of mine squeaks and aches when it moves, making me. Do I have to learn to walk and talk and breathe in the world differently? Am I brave enough to try?

The Xanax bottle ended up in my purse, my blood in a small colony of vials (results almost shockingly normal), and supplements called "Tropical Breeze Calming Effect" and "Somno-Pro" in my mouth, with no effect that I could actually discern. I found myself both disappointed and slightly smug about that. What, you think you know me better than me? Ha! Also, I sort of wish you did.

I forced myself back into the Witch Doctor's lair. The hippie pills didn't work, what else do you have? How much more disappointment can I swallow before I give in?

She frowned—not at me, for she is a good witch—paused a minute, and let the gears click into place in her head. "We're going to pull out the big guns for you."

I braced myself for the verdict: Lexapro? Celexa? Klonopin? Valium? A friend told me recently of a mild antipsychotic that had sufficiently ball-gagged his inner demons. How much collateral damage would I incur this time to silence mine?

Next weapon in her arsenal: L-theanine. It's an amino acid derived from tea leaves and, she swore, more effective in blind clinical trials than Xanax. In fact, she said, "Think of it as natural Xanax—one that you'll actually let yourself take." (I was fooling no one.) "You can get it on the Internet, but from what I can see, you need relief NOW. Go to the front desk and book our next appointment, then go to the health food store. Two hundred milligrams to start. GO."

I dawdled a little. I'll admit that. As eager as I was to stop picking and grinding (I could probably haul a semi with my jaw for at least a couple of exits at this point, it gets such a constant workout), it just seemed stupid to hope. I stopped into a GNC on my way to the office, shuddered at the price of the house brand, and put off my mission. Over the course of the next few days, I found more excuses until I eventually ran out of them. I slunk into the holistisustaina-locaganivore market a few blocks from my home and scoured the shelves of elfsbane, pixiewort, mermaid tusk, and weird, random beans until I found the "relaxation" section. Holy hell, was it big. If I hadn't been sweatily clutching a scrap of paper with the name, brand, and dosage like a character in a Christopher Nolan film, I'd have run screaming into the street. I bought it, though. Bought it and took it, and I'm terrified to say . . . I think it's helping. My hands would probably be quivering typing these words had I not just popped a tiny dose to quell a panic attack I felt rising up. I'm cautious with taking it—treating my brain like a frightened pet bunny, sneaking gently, slowly up to soothe it. L-theanine thus far . . . *thus far* . . . isn't any sort of blanket, cloud, or shroud for my fitful brain. Doesn't muffle, just strokes and smooths the jagged-edged thoughts like I'm getting a brain massage. (Which is a weird thing for me to enjoy, because massages tend to freak me the hell out.)

It doesn't make me feel anything extra—just less bothered by it all, and only sometimes, but I'll take it. I'm afraid to even form these words, have these notions, because it will just jinx everything (apparently L-theanine does nothing to quell magical thinking). I'm afraid that I'll relax and have all the calm snatched back because it is not what I'm supposed to get.

A friend was laughing at me tonight when I told him about my quandary. "You're anxious about something that relieves anxiety? This is the Kat Kinsman I know and love!" he wrote to me, but that's just it. If I'm not bracing for the next bad thing, how will I be ready when it comes?

IRRATIONAL FEAR #6
HAVING CHILDREN

When we were ten, my friend Mary told me that I'd make a terrible mother, and while I protested aloud at the time, deep down I had to agree with her at least a little. The crux of her argument was that because I told her if it had been me whose social studies project had been pulled off the shelf and mangled by my mother's home daycare kids (whose diapers I had to change even though they weren't my siblings *and* I wasn't getting paid), I'd be mad as HE-double-hockey-sticks, I just didn't understand what it was like to love children.

In retrospect, I imagine she was suffering from a touch of Stockholm syndrome—which most people might find a useful coping mechanism in the midst of a few dozen, non-blood-related, shrieking infants and toddlers—but she was my friend and it hurt my feelings. Perhaps I hadn't articulated it clearly enough (ten-year-old girls often don't), but what I was trying to get across was that I was worried about her and frankly offended by the injustice done to her in her own home. This social studies project was a great big percentage of our grade for the quarter, and I couldn't imagine her having to go in and explain that she had finished the articulated

3-D map and everything, but it was now in a billion soggy scraps at the bottom of a garbage can. My stomach ached on her behalf, but she just seemed to take it in stride. "God, Katie, that's just what little kids do. What's wrong with you?"

A fair question, and one that even at that early age, I asked myself a lot. Other girls and even a few of the boys seemed to relish the feeding, mopping, and battery-powered mewling of realistic baby dolls, role-playing a version of adulthood centered around keeping a creature dry and quiet. I wondered why they'd voluntarily invite that kind of stress into their lives. Didn't they see how kids were a problem—how we were a problem? So far as I could tell, or for as far back as I could remember, my sister and I were a source of unrest to our parents. Whether it was worrying about our whereabouts and safety, if we were being preyed on by adult men with bad intentions or rude boys who wanted to teach us the word "fart," if we were squabbling with each other, making noise of any kind, or wasting the day inside and unproductive rather than doing something with ourselves, we were causing them to worry. Or, rather, causing Mumsie to worry, which caused Pup to worry, which caused him to have to comfort her and correct us (quite loudly sometimes)—which made me worried for me and for the agita I was clearly inflicting on their lives and . . . God, why did anyone have kids in the first place? I didn't feel unloved, but definitely like a strain on my parents' well-being, and maybe that's what love was after all: constant fret about the condition of the people you bring into this world. Love means never getting to say, "No big whoop."

I felt bad for Mary. Her mother clearly didn't care as much as mine because she took it all in stride, offering little sympathy for her daughter's plight, suggesting she might have put it on a higher shelf or in her room if she meant to keep it safe. It didn't occur to me that her mom maintained this home daycare business because she was genuinely gifted at tending to little ones and that it allowed other parents to go about their workday calm in the knowledge that their beloved offspring were in safe and happy hands. Or that she did this so that her own children could have a roof over their heads, new clothes, and enough to eat. It just seemed to me like an infliction of noise, chaos, and a million potential crises into what could have been a peaceful home.

My perspective has shifted over the years, of course, broadened beyond worry as a benchmark for loving someone—but the notion of motherhood still scares the hell out of me. I cannot have children of my own because I am afraid of raising them to be afraid, and I am no longer young enough to change my mind anyway. It would be easy for someone to interpret this as the dislike of kids. They do so all the time with women like me who are childless by choice—and some of those women probably do dislike kids—but in my case, they're incorrect. I love the weird kids, the ones who don't naturally slide into their assigned place in the world, assured that it's all theirs for the making and taking. It meant the world to me to see odd adults thriving in the world, and it meant everything when they took time to actually see me and treat me like a human rather than a nuisance. I try to do the same.

I know firsthand and painfully what it is like to be the child of someone who suffers from severe anxiety, cannot control it, or even always articulate it. How your life becomes about the maintenance of someone else's mood, and to know that you are often the root cause—not because of anything you did, necessarily, but just because you exist. How you learn to watch your words, mute yourself, and blunt your angles so as not to ratchet up their suffering.

Researchers have yet to prove a hereditary predisposition toward anxiety, but really, it barely matters. Just as a child learns to speak, eat, dress, brush their teeth, ride a bike and comb their hair, they learn to flinch at a ringing phone, cower from sirens, quadruple-check the iron, and hold their breath while driving, all by watching their parents. Anxiety, even well maintained, ripples outward, and the people around you learn to bob in its wake so they won't drown.

I knew, even back then, that I couldn't do that to a child. Call it selfish if you insist, but to me, it's a kindness not to replicate my searing gut, my shaking hands, my thrumming pulse, airless lungs, and sleepless nights. I can't inflict that physical hell and mental torment on an innocent soul. And I know with every quivering fiber of my being that if I gave birth to a daughter or son, I would not be at rest for one second unless I knew she or he was right in front of me, safe and sound. That's no way to let a life grow and flourish, so I don't. I can't. I won't.

The use of birth control is almost pathological for me, and my decision not to have children factored massively into my dating life. By my late twenties, while it wasn't the first thing I led with while getting to know someone new (Hi, I'm Kat. I'm a Leo who loves bourbon, Nabokov, collard greens, and the color red, and by the way, any chance you've had a vasectomy?), if I found myself in profound like with someone (i.e., considering sleeping with them), I made it abundantly clear that "Oh, baby!" wasn't ever going to take on deeper meaning for me.

I used to wonder if there was something broken in me—other than the anxiety and depression, I mean—that I didn't feel some grand pang or push toward motherhood, but rather the opposite. I've seen my friends become mothers, grandmothers, even. Most of their daughters and sons have been born healthy and stayed that way, others have had knots and rips from the start or along the way.

Some have traveled overseas to meet their children who may not be of their blood but who have all their heart and others have married and melded their families. I knelt by my best friend Beannie's side, held her head in my hand and her knee in the crook of my arm, while she gritted her teeth and pushed out her son. I watched her face transform as she stared into his eyes for the first time, love metamorphosing her into a mother, and it remains one of the most wondrous things I have ever had the privilege to behold.

I'll never know that particular joy in my lifetime. And I'm oddly at peace with it.

IRRATIONAL FEAR #7
ALTERNATIVE REMEDIES

The next time someone asks me if I have heard of mindfulness, I am going to ask them to try a small exercise with me. We will face one another at arm's length, stand still, and lower our eyelids. Then, when I am confident we have both done so, I will open mine, reach out, and flick them once, solidly, at the center of their forehead so they can be fully present for it. Yes, of course I have heard of mindfulness. And meditation of various flavors and yoga and prayer and massage and kava and cognitive behavioral therapy and GABA supplements and weed edibles and that app your cousin worked on. I am at this point a professional anxious-ologist, and if it exists as a potential mitigator of anxiety, I have if not tried it, at least clocked some serious study hours. (Notice I said "mitigator of" rather than "cure for" because that's a hell of a lot of pressure to put on any given technique or substance, when anxiety is pretty much an auto-immune disease of the soul.) I thoroughly appreciate that people want to share a solution that has been effective for themselves or a loved one. If you are at all a sensitive person, you see another crea-ture in pain and you want to heal it. But if there is one thing I have learned in all my years battling this feral cat in private and public, it's that while different things work well for different people, there is no panacea. And it can start to feel grueling and frustrating—and indeed anxiety-inducing—to run headlong toward a technique, only to have the possibility of relief yanked away from you like Charlie Brown and the football. You begin to feel un-calmable and that's not calming at all.

For what it's worth, what's worked for me thus far in my four decades of more or less constant fret: Cognitive Behavioral Therapy paired with the occasional bit of hypnosis, taking series of three deep breaths through my nose and out of my mouth, walking on the treadmill while listening to Kanye West, watching *Mad Max: Fury Road*, holding Douglas's hand, saying the alphabet in my head repeatedly until I forget why I'm upset, orgasms, Champagne, L-theanine, petting my animals, walking through Chinatown, riding Ferris wheels, and that's pretty much it. Anything else either causes anxiety—or at least does little to quell it. It's okay and I've learned to live with that low-level sour soul buzz, but I can't go around getting overly jazzed about the potential efficacy of a treatment and I can't be well for the sake of someone else, even if they mean so very well.

The last yoga class I took was at Douglas's behest. He was worried about me, and with good reason. For several weeks, my anxiety had been in an especially violent spiral, whipping me past any respite I tried to reach out and grab. Sleep? Not a chance. If I'd finally manage to collapse from sheer exhaustion, before two hours were up I'd be shocked awake by stress dreams and the hammer of my heartbeat.

Medication? Yeah, maybe—if the prospect of locating a potential new physician and (ohgodohgodohgod) picking up the phone to call to see if they were taking new patients weren't so very daunting. And it would have been great to chat it out with my therapist of fifteen years—if he hadn't abruptly stopped his practice after a mysterious "medical incident" a few months before. I'd held out hope, but he wasn't coming back and I wasn't getting any calmer, and dammit—I guess I'm doing this. But please come with me to assure that I make it through the door.

We turned out to be the only two people who felt spiritually drawn to a beginner-level "calming" class that Monday evening, so we had the full benefit of guidance by the earnest, rubber-band-bodied healer who gave us her card, redeemable for 15 percent off a couples bodywork session on side-by-side suspended jade tables at her other practice, which was not at the Ninth Street YMCA.

"Thank you," I said, tucking it into my moisture-wicking sports bra. "We will think about that."

It was all very generous of her, this combination meditation/yoga instruction in the moist, bleach-swabbed exercise room. I know this because she kept telling us about the gift of calm she was bestowing upon our agitated minds and bodies. After a few preliminary stretches and breaths that I utterly failed to execute with any acceptable degree of serenity. ("You know you carry your tension in your neck and shoulders? Have you tried relaxing them?" "What, and lose this alluring Marty Feldman posture I've worked so hard to master? I'll get right on that.") Guru Jade Table invited us to assume corpse pose uponst our borrowed mats.

"You just kinda lie on your back," I whispered to Douglas, who'd never done yoga before and, as far as I could intuit from his rolling eyes, would not be making a steady practice of it.

I tried. Oh, I tried so kicking, screaming, bleeding hard to let the stress leach from my body to the mat, through the floor, into the subbasement down to trickle onto the subway train rumbling below. I tried to envision the overflow of my upsets and concerns flowing down into the squishy, purple mat and dissolving—psssh!—into the psychic landfill. But maybe mine was defective, or thoroughly sodden with the emotional backwash of the thousands of spiritual pilgrims who passed through this sacred gymnasium before me. Because it started to soak back in, and ohm shanti, did it sting. I could hear my pulse in my ears and feel each separate sizzle of muscle fiber, screaming to be set back into motion so I could escape.

Stripped of the distraction of movement, sound, and speech, I was suddenly acutely aware of the hornets' swarm of thoughts that now had room to move freely about the cabin. They echoed across the emptiness: "billlzzzzz . . . deadlinezzzz . . . dizzzappointment of friendzzzz . . . wow, do youzzz zzzuuuuck at zzzziiiizzz . . ."

"Shhh!" I whispered to the buzzing horde. "Just let me have this moment. This is supposed to be my time to be free of all of this. To achieve calm. Wait . . . why aren't I achieving calm? Calm down, what's wrong with you? ACHIEVE DIVINE CALM, FOR KRISHNA'S SAKE!"

But neither Krishna nor any of the other major or minor deities were taking calls from skeptical, lapsed-Catholic girls in YMCA fitness rooms that day—unless they were the ones stretching the seconds and minutes to ten times their length in some sort of trickster-god lesson in infinite patience.

Oh, who was I trying to kid? It wasn't any sort of cosmic prank or the fault of the gods or of an age-old spiritual practice into which I was naively and arrogantly sticking my little toe. It surely was not the fault of Guru Jade Table, who truly was generously presenting me with the gift of her years of study. I was just too much of a trembling dope to know how to unwrap it.

This particular moment of enlightenment, humbling as it was, did not suddenly allow my tensed muscle fibers and pinging neural pathways to soften and flood with calm. Nope—pretty much the opposite.

If I couldn't find a modicum of bliss and relief in something that had stilled millions of souls throughout the millennia, it was distinctly possible that I was clinically un-calmable. Great—a whole new thing to worry about.

So I lay there in silence and agony, stomach roiling, pulse jack-hammering, jaw clenched, and muscles tensing by the second. I resisted opening my eyes for fear of failing the exercise even more deeply, but I could have sworn that Guru Jade Table had actually left and forgotten about us, it had been so long since she'd spoken aloud.

We'd gotten there on a Monday around eight o'clock or so—it had to be at least Thursday afternoon by now, and I'd missed most of the workweek and I'd probably been fired. Our dogs were likely starving and/or dead. The rabbit, too. And our apartment probably burned down, of course that's what that passing siren was. Stupid, careless, selfish me for leaving home—or bed, for that matter.

I grasped wildly for some sort of sensory indicator that would anchor me to the here and now. Okay, another subway train rumbling under us, so that means at least seven minutes have passed since the last one—or is it twelve? Is it a holiday schedule today? Is that thunder or did someone tip a set of barbells in the weight room upstairs? Did I die from a panic attack? Am I dead? If I'd known I was headed to the afterlife straight from the gym, I'd have worn something more appropriate than these leggings with the blingy rhinestone skull. But then again . . .

And suddenly it pierced through the crackling chaos, clear as a wolf whistle and as familiar to me as the burned-in scar on my right forearm: Douglas's sleep breathing. He wasn't yet at a full-fledged snore, but he'd hit the wall and slumped against it. His day begins at 5:20 A.M. and roller-coaster careens through until at least 7 P.M. After that, the briefest break in pace trips his off switch and he's out.

I envy my husband this, and I figured he wouldn't mind if I borrowed a pinch of his repose. I willed my body to match its breath to his, echo its rise and release. For about forty-five glorious seconds, it worked. I was free. I was mildly less nauseatingly stressed out since I'd lain down on the communal gym mat that evening, and maybe that's just as tranquil as it gets for me. I am at one with that possibility. I give myself over to the divine Ninth Street YMCA deities. I . . . crap.

Time to stand up and stretch—another exercise in humiliation for me. Despite the recent knee surgery and lack of a functioning anterior cruciate ligament, my graceful, groggy husband is a former dancer whose muscles and tendons vividly recall thousands of hours of barre exercises and grand arabesques and whatnot. I'd been a high school cheerleader who went to art school to double-major in cross-legged brooding and wild gesticulation. Graceful flexibility: not so much my forte.

"Reeelaaaaax your neck muscles. Feel your head dripping toward the floor. Let your shoulders go."

I stole a glance over at Douglas, who so far as I could tell had gotten his skeletal system surgically replaced by Silly Putty in the last few minutes. I tried to suffuse my soul with delight at his ability to so successfully chillax. I failed.

Jade sidled over. "Maybe we'll try something else for you."

I wobbled my head on its creaky hinge. Yes, let's do that.

The last thing I could take at this point was to feel as if I'd failed another person who'd been kind enough to try to help me. Yes, she was being compensated for her efforts, and it wasn't as if the

Y was going to snip a chunk out of her check because one of her students failed to transcend her corporeal inhibitions. But she was a stranger who cared enough to try, and for that, I owed her. Owed her a day when she didn't feel a little bit worse about herself than when she'd woken up and saluted the sun. I couldn't have that on my conscience.

So I lied. I let her lead me through the nose-inhaling, arm-pumping breathing exercise she proudly proclaimed had knocked a few hundred Ground Zero rescuers out of a cycle of debilitating panic attacks after 9/11. I hadn't mentioned that I'd incurred a small panic attack during nighty-night time on the yoga mat, but it didn't take Deepak Chopra to be attuned to the psychic lightning storm that was zapping inside my clench-molared head.

I gave it my snuffling, snotty all, doing my best to crumple my upset into a ball and exorcise it through my nasal passages, jotting a mental note to bring a yoga mat the next time. After I shopped for a yoga mat.

If Jade's intent was to short-circuit the anxiety loop by inducing hyperventilation-induced euphoria, mission accomplished. But for a pulse already at a fluttering hummingbird pace, this fell just short of disastrous—swirling high-grade cocaine into the nectar feeder.

But it wasn't her fault. She was a kind woman who carried around a tool kit that just didn't fit my broken parts. I wasn't sure that the correct one existed on this mortal plane or any beyond, so, you know, A for effort. *Danke schoen, merci,* and *namaste,* Guru Jade Table.

And when she asked if I felt better, I lied, like I have to countless therapists, family members, lovers, friends, and so many well-meaning people who have offered me care and calm. Did this massage make you feel better? This chat, this tea, this kiss? Yes, thank you. You are so kind and I appreciate it more than you know. (That last part is true.) They had no idea what they were up against—armed with a popgun when it would take a howitzer to blast through my walls. And God help 'em if they see what's on the other side.

But I don't lie to Douglas. I never have and I've never tried. If anything, I tried to scare him off right up front by letting him know what he was up against, both for his sake and for mine. I didn't want to draw him into my spiral when I knew he couldn't slow it, and I didn't want to lean and rest against a shoulder that would slip away from the force of my spinning, unquiet mind. I warned him—I did—telling him look, I've seen therapists for over half my life. I take pills to keep my brain from screaming. I fall down into dank, dark pits, and you cannot pull me out. There is no fixing me, and it's not your job and you might as well know that right up front.

"Try me," he said. And I did.

And as we slipped on our shoes and trudged up the hill toward our apartment, he asked me, "Did that help?"

"Nah," I sighed.

And he squeezed my hand. That helped a little bit.

CHAPTER NINE

Home Is Where the Fear Hides

"'You've been in the house too long,' she said, and I naturally fled."

At thirty-three, I was still living in the fifth-floor, rent-stabilized walk-up apartment where I'd crash-landed in an acquaintance's newly spare bedroom after our mutual friends decided that I needed to vacate the grimy, moldy, illegal, unheated warehouse in front of which I'd been mugged of my last seven dollars by a group of seven teenagers. The acquaintance eventually moved in with her boyfriend and I'd had the place to myself for a good chunk of the eight years I'd lived there, but I'd never really bothered to unpack.

That would only jinx things, I told myself. Why should I assume that I was being granted some measure of stability? This was my fourth address since moving to Brooklyn nearly a decade before, and I still hadn't eased myself free of the quiver I felt every time I passed my landlord's apartment door on the second floor. Ralph hadn't been thrilled to find that Tami, the person on the lease, had taken on a roommate, and was even less delighted to find I'd stayed behind after she'd vanished. Still, he figured, letting me stay (at a modest rent increase) was cheaper for him than having to paint the place, upgrade the cold-war-era fridge, and make the radiators produce the occasional wisp of heat along with their freight-train clamor—all of which he'd have to do to attract a new tenant.

This was both an ideal and awful place for an anxious person to live. The apartment spanned the whole length of the left side of the building, from a front room that dangled above a noisy Brooklyn avenue to a kitchen fire escape that I could have clambered down to the weedy, ratty, fenced-in backyard below but of course never did. Deep in the center, I hid from the world.

The bedroom that had been assigned to me when I moved in was a small, windowless, airless cube with a sticky linoleum floor and an unfortunate acoustic tic that channeled all the creaks and moans from the couple below directly upward. Once I learned to block that out (along with the shrieks of the infant that eventually resulted from all that bumping in the night), that room became my haven—and something of a hovel.

I lived like a feral thing in there, creeping out and playing at being a human from time to time, and then scurrying back in to protect myself from the world and vice versa. Tami and I got along just fine, but I was all too aware that she'd done me a kindness by letting me move into her spare room, and that the favor could be rescinded at any time. Before the warehouse, I had been housed with a thirty-five-year-old art student who'd come to her senses and begged her mother for funds so she wouldn't have to split the rent with a slobby twenty-five-year-old who hogged the phone line with her dial-up modem and was always late with her half of the gas bill. (I didn't blame her—I wouldn't have wanted to live with me either.) And before that, I'd suddenly found myself persona non grata in my own home for having the gall to suggest that my roommate's visiting (and, I slowly came to realize, live-in) boyfriend occasionally bother to lock the apartment door so we wouldn't get robbed, murdered, assaulted, and whatnot in our first Brooklyn apartment after grad school.

Opening my mouth then made living in the place that was (so far as my bank account was concerned) my home had cost me, so I now made as light and compact a residential footprint as I could. It was the only way I knew how to survive.

If there had been one defining rule in my home growing up, it was this: don't disturb your mother once she has calmed down enough to rest. It is wrong. It is mean. There will be hell to pay.

I understand now that her outbursts and accusations, random jags of howling sobs and wails—all stemmed from a brain and body that were out of balance. When Pup would corral her into the den and shut the door, to soothe her and muffle her shrieks, it wasn't because I'd committed a mortal sin by galumphing up the stairs too loudly, getting a phone call after she'd lain down for a nap, or leaving my book bag on the table. Even if she'd said it was.

I know that now, but back then, I believed I'd broken her by having the audacity to exist. Once Pup had filed down the edges of my mother's agitation and shepherded her spent body onto the couch or into bed, by God, the rest of us had better shut the hell up.

Again, I know now how little sense that makes, that someone who's attached their heart to yours would suddenly snap that connection just because you've broken a glass or woken them up with a creak on the stairs. Annoyance and upset, sure. But real love isn't that conditional and a loud thump (likely) won't get you cast out onto the street.

I wish I could whisper that to shuddering six-year-old me who'd taken my mother's words to heart when she'd calmly, coldly told my sister and me that our fairly frequent, screaming fights had sparked some discussion between her and Pup. "We're very seriously considering putting the two of you up for adoption if you don't learn how to get along and play nicely together. We are just tired of it and we don't want our lives to be like this."

She went back to her ironing and my sister and I stared at each other in shock. We were used to getting scolded for our squabbles, but this felt different, like the ground beneath our home had shifted.

I might have been able to slough it off, tap-dance and sparkle to show my mother I loved her extra-vibrantly so it would be harder for her to cast me away, but I looked over at my sister, who was starting to shake and cry. My sister, who was made of much tougher stuff than I was and who gave no obvious damn about our mother's affection, believed what she'd heard. The two of us never touched except in anger, but we instinctively lunged into each other's arms and babbled out our apologies.

"We'll be good, we promise. We'll get along. We'll play nice. We'll be quiet. We'll be good. We'll be good. Don't give us away."

Our parents were kind enough to keep us on staff (I asked Pup about it a few years back and I was thoroughly un-shocked to find out that they'd had no discussion of the sort, and she'd never told him about the incident), but there was something about that particular exchange, out of her billion unintentional weirdnesses over the years, that took root and wound around some part of my brain that rationally processed how this whole loving/being loved thing works.

If anything, it emboldened my sister to kick and beat her fists at the boundaries. Her act became "I'm loud—do you love me now? I'll walk ten steps in front of the family pretending I don't know you, do you still love me? I'll sulk in the car, threatening to run away, scowling in family photographs, skipping dinner, saying no, no, NO to all of you. I belong to you whether you want me to or not."

And I crouched down, afraid to move or make a sound. Tami,

her boyfriend, and her two elderly, incontinent, yowling cats had the run of the apartment and did so at full and lusty volume. They (the humans, not the cats) wrote songs for their band, threw spontaneous two-person dance parties, ordered mountains of pizzas and fries that grew cold in their open boxes (and never quite made it to the trash can), squabbled and cooed loudly on the phone, and went about the business of being in their twenties in then-inexpensive Brooklyn. I stayed in my room, afraid that if the universe noticed me, the great, cosmic Whac-A-Mole that had bopped me down before would come cracking down on my skull again. I ate in my room. I worked in my room. I talked on the phone, watched TV, read books, wrote letters, listened to music, broke up with my long-distance boyfriend, and slept endless, undisturbed hours in that safe, still place, growing ever more afraid of the world outside it.

Even after Tami moved out, I didn't treat the rest of the apartment as a place to live. I just sort of haunted it, afraid that if I made my presence known in a way that disturbed a single soul, I'd be exorcised. When I ran into one of the downstairs loud-humpers a few months into my solo tenancy, she was shocked to find that we hadn't both moved out. "We thought the apartment was just sitting there empty," she told me. "That would explain a lot," I didn't say out loud.

I found myself oddly proud of my perch as the seldom seen, rarely heard upstairs neighbor. Tucked away on the top floor, I hovered above the bustle and hunger of the world below and bothered no one save for the occasional required foray.

In lieu of making noise, I make a mess. It's a thing I have always done, and that I simply loathe about myself, but somehow can't seem to rein in. It's a shameful thing, being a messy person, and I try to minimize the spillover into other people's lives. Maybe it started as an act of rebellion, parallel to my sister's clattering double-dog-dare. If she could stomp and yell, I could stack and strew, and if I kept the clutter behind my own closed doors, it wasn't technically bothering anyone. It was within the rules, so they still had to love me. But they were family and they had to.

Soon after my boyfriend of two and a half years broke up with me, for reasons that surely included the way I lived in my mess of an apartment, I lost another reason to enter the outside world. I had been working as an online art director at a magazine, and budget cuts lopped off almost every job in my department. While I was lucky enough to pick up a fantastic new gig as the webmistress of the Yoo-hoo chocolate drink website (yes, that's an actual job and it was mine for a very long time), after a few panicky weeks, I realized it didn't entail physically having to be anywhere. Talking to anyone. Leaving my home. Manifesting in front of anyone. So long as the work showed up online, it didn't matter if it was posted from Anchorage or Angola, Zanzibar or Zimbabwe. I could have traveled the world as long as I posted regularly. Of course, all the posts emanated from a dark, cluttered, quiet cave in Brooklyn.

After the initial shock of the September 11 attack on New York City (my third day at this wondrous new job), my friends first clung together and then the couples cleaved to themselves to mourn and heal. I tried to be of as much use as I could, sending bundles of socks and handwritten thank-you cards to first responders, checking in on friends and sobbing strangers (and buying them lots and lots and lots of drinks), hugging random firefighters, and trying repeatedly to give blood (it turned out very little was needed), and when it turned out there wasn't a whole lot I could actually do, I removed myself from the equation.

I had plenty of time to hide myself. Not long before the attack,

I'd gone on a few dates with John, a cute, wry, and unserious fellow who worked in the financial district. He posed no real threat to my heart, but was awfully fun to make out with on street corners. I liked that he wore a tie—if messily—in the off-hours, and was learning to play the accordion. So far as I could tell, he was impressed that I'd used to work at his favorite men's magazine and knew more than him about cocktails. On September 5, 2001, we stopped at an ATM near his office to each get cash before seeing an early-evening showing of *Jay and Silent Bob Strike Back* (not my choice, but early in a relationship I liked to show what a good sport I was). I tilted my head as far back as it would go, staring up into the sharp glare of the late-summer sky.

"What do you think would happen if one of these fell?" I wondered aloud.

"Wellll . . . ," he mused, "it would probably screw up traffic downtown for a pretty long time."

September 8, 2001, he and I kissed on a picnic blanket atop the lush jade grass of Manhattan's Battery Park.

Three days later, that lawn was strewn with ash and rubble, and John and I were volleying short, frantic e-mails back and forth.

"Oh God, where are you? Are you in the office?"

"I don't know what's happening. They won't tell us anything."

"What are you seeing? Can you get out of there?"

"I can see people jumping out the window. They're just falling out onto the sidewalk."

"Go go go go go. Get out of there. GET OUT OF THERE! Stay safe and let me know when you're home, please? I'll try to find out more. Just get out of there."

John walked home, all the way from his office in the bank headquarters across from the World Trade Center to his apartment in

Astoria, Queens, up through Manhattan and over the Fifty-ninth Street Bridge, mostly in his socks because his brand-new dress shoes were still stiff and blistered his feet. I tried to keep in touch with him, but it was hard once he decided he needed to move back in with his parents on Long Island for a few months. I certainly didn't blame him for needing to curl up and be someone's child again for a little while.

With no significant other, nearby family, set work hours, or office to get to, it was probably easy to miss the fact that I was disappearing. I didn't mind—the fewer people who worried about me, the less guilt I had about taxing their strained resources. For those over whom I was watching, I did my best to be a present, warm, bulletproof blanket that could absorb any residual terror they were feeling, but from afar as much as possible.

In late 2001, in New York City, there was no "normal," just a general acceptance that whatever you were doing to cope was pretty much A-OK. Eating nothing but grilled cheese or having a blood-alcohol level of .08 at all times? You just take care of you, baby. Popping Xanax like Tic Tacs, bunking down with pretty strangers, or taking a one-way cab ride back home to the Midwest? Not unheard of, and surely not judged by anyone with a zip code in the five boroughs or right across the Hudson. If a friend seemed fairly free of twitches, random new habits, phobias, or periodic crying jags, the consensus was that she or he just hadn't gotten around to processing things yet.

I gave a good impression of what passed for okay, I thought. My friend Lissa and I flew defiantly, frequently (and cheaply) to Las Vegas in the ensuing months, declaring that if the bad guys were going to get us, they might as well take us down in the epicenter of excess. Round-trip tickets on a now-defunct casino-owned airline were eighty-six dollars, rooms at the Flamingo were fifty-three dollars a night (with the third night free, so might as well stay that—or six), and dammit, we were doing our patriotic duty by double-tipping for drinks and meals when the tourist industry crawled to a halt. We learned quickly when it was safe to cop to being from New York (mostly to other New Yorkers) and when to demur to our childhood hometowns to avoid the sharp hiss of breath through the teeth and "Oooohhh . . . I'm sorry."

We drank. We rode mechanical bulls. We bet the next round on which escort would first exit the premises with a conventioneer in pleated khakis and a cell-phone holster. We danced sweatily with strangers. We came home late, slept into the afternoon, and slapped cheap pancakes, massive omelets, and hash browns atop our hangovers. Lissa lounged by the pool reading Elmore Leonard novels and biographies of Maria Callas while I hunched over a laptop in our room to do the work that funded my sojourns from reality.

If you've never been to Las Vegas (and are not in the habit of gambling, which, luckily, I never have been), despite the veil of debauchery, it can be a surprisingly effective place to take a break from the burden of being a person. Not from being mindful of the feelings and well-being of one's fellow humans, 'cause that's never cool, but a main street boasting a sphinx, a half-size Eiffel Tower, a man-made lake, and a semi-nightly pirate battle is a pretty solid indicator that you don't have to be at work in the morning.

I deeply dreaded coming home each time, even though the apartment was my safe haven. It was the getting inside that nearly killed me. There was the stomach stinging and pulse crashing in the hollow of my throat as the cab pulled off the Brooklyn–Queens Expressway, left on Flatbush, right on Fourth Avenue, left on Union—no, the corner is fine, thanks, I just need to get my bag from the trunk. With the first glimpse of my building's scarred, harvest-orange door, the panic locomotive started.

Okay. Okay. Building is still standing. Good. That means I didn't leave the stove on and burn the place down. Whew. Was worried. Victory number two—key works in the front door, so Ralph hasn't evicted me for . . . I dunno what. Something. Something bad I did, or forgot to do. Next hurdle . . . oh God, oh God, what's come in the mail. Maybe the eviction notice is there. Or a bill I forgot to pay. Or final warning on . . . something, the universe, yes, the universe telling me that I suck and everyone knows it. Or maybe that a relative has died. Maybe Mumsie died and everyone forgot my cell phone number and they don't have my e-mail address and this is how they're telling me. Oh, whew—just the gas bill. I'll pay that. Okay, I hope Ralph won't hear me lugging my suitcase up the stairs. He'll want to ask me how I am and want to hug me and I just . . . I just can't right now. Whew . . . made it. One more flight to go aaaand, thank goodness, my key still works. I still live here. OH MY GOD, the light isn't turning on, did the electricity get turned off?! Oh . . . just a burned-out bulb. I'll ask Ralph to bring his ladder and fix it . . . but I have to clean up the hallway first so he doesn't see how awful I've let the place get. I'll do that tomorrow, I just need to sit down for a little while.

That bulb stayed burned out for a very long time.

I don't quite remember how or when I completely stopped going down the stairs during the daytime, or letting people come into my apartment. Way up in my fifth-floor perch, I was still able to drink my fill of the sun by spending endless hours fussing over various tomato-plant crises on the rickety, red fire escape, or hauling two-liter bottles of water up to the silver-sealed rooftop in a futile attempt to keep the cornstalks and pumpkin vines I was growing there from withering to dust. That never quite worked, but I didn't stop trying.

In the years before texts, Twitter, FaceTime, Facebook, and Skype's constant pawing and demanding instant acknowledgment, it was easier to give the impression of someone who operated on a semi-human schedule. Send out a barrage of e-mails in the early-morning hours before sleep, hop on conference calls at the mandated times, show up late for the evening's dinner plans with a breathless excuse about a stalled train—it was easy to keep up the illusion that I was hunky-dory, A-OK, peachy keen, and a functional member of society. I got my work done (though mostly in the middle of the night), met my deadlines, showed up in cute shoes with lipstick on to meet my friends, and no one had any idea what it cost me to get there.

Somehow, my front door became impassable before the sun went down. Didn't matter if I was fading from a blood sugar crash and had no food in the house, the post office was about to close, or my friends were at the restaurant waiting for me, the prospect of releasing the chain, grabbing the handle, stepping through the door frame, and tottering down all five floors simply undid me. The minute I'd step into the bathroom to brush my teeth and smear on makeup, my hands would begin to shake so badly sometimes that I'd foul up my task (usually the eyeliner, but there were an awful lot of dropped toothpaste caps), have to wash my face, and start all over again with my heart racing and my throat constricting and oh, crap . . . I'm going to be late AGAIN. Dammit. And sure, I could have left my house looking like an unmade bed, but then everyone would know that something was amiss. Now where are my shoes? Ah, over there by that teetering pile of papers, and stupid me . . . I shouldn't have left that glass of Diet Coke there where I *knew* it would get knocked over. I get so clumsy when I'm stressed, and is it hot in here? I'm burning up and now I'm sure there are sweat stains on this dress and I can't let anyone see me like this. I can't let anyone see me . . .

And they didn't. Not like that.

There's a pat, smug bit of "wisdom" that people like to parrot—that those who are always late are doing so out of arrogance, because they think that nothing important could possibly happen before they arrived. Nope.

For a lot of us who deal with anxiety and panic, it can be an act of courage and will to approach the front door and walk through it. The thought of leaving your little cocoon—be it whatever level of fancy or humble, neat as a pin or as messy as a hoarder's hovel—can be paralyzing, and that's completely mortifying. Millions, BILLIONS of people walk out their front door, baby on hip, cell phone glued to ear, purse on shoulder, armed for entrée into the world, and thoroughly unencumbered by angst. For them, and I'm just guessing here, the door just works one way, depending on what side of it they're on. It keeps the world at bay when they're inside, and beckons them back in upon their return. Easy peasy.

But for me, that door felt bolstered by the force of the universe pressing in and sealing me in to starve and crumble. To leave meant I had to shore up all my strength for many minutes, sometimes hours, and sometimes days, to throw myself against it and burst out into the bright, raw daylight of my neighborhood, where someone I knew might see me and ask me how I was (in Vegas, that was a near-statistical impossibility). And I wasn't in the clear once I made it over my threshold either. There were still five floors' worth of stairs to contend with, and no guarantee that my knees would be able to complete their assigned task either.

Sometimes the pep talk worked. I'd make it down to the sidewalk, slink to whatever store was still open, and stock up on as much

Diet Coke, toilet paper, single-serve brownies, green grapes, tortilla chips, hummus, soy milk, and Barbara's Peanut Butter Puffins as I could possibly fit in my arms, knowing that it might be a while before I could risk getting the bends from the descent. Other times, I'd mete out my self-reward with a single liter of Diet Coke and a turkey-and-Swiss sandwich rather than stocking up on provisions, so I'd be forced to return to street level again.

And every once in a while, I'd burst through the air lock before dusk fell, break free of the building's magnetic pull, and sprint to freedom. Those were the days I'd send up a flare to the people I loved and missed. "Hey, I'm out running around, want to grab a bite?" And it would turn into an evening.

"Should we call so-and-so?"

"Oh, that would be great! I haven't seen her in ages!"

"I haven't seen YOU in ages! Is work just crazy busy?"

"Work is just sooooooo crazy busy. I feel like I haven't seen me in forever either. Tell me all about youuuuuuuu . . ."

"OMG, I have so much to tell you. And so-and-so just said she'd bring so-and-so, is that cool?"

"Totally! Let's see if we can grab one of these big tables . . ."

If you can seem shiny and happy in front of a large group of people at once, you have witnesses and they will spread the word to the rest of the world. "Oh, I just saw her a couple of weeks ago. She seemed great!" And you're off the hook for a while, and probably a little exhausted.

It takes work to shoulder the burden of everyone's concern, and I did my best to minimize it during my visits to ground level, because I certainly wasn't going to let anyone up to see how I was living.

After the breakup with Sam, it felt increasingly possible that I could close the door to my apartment and slowly fade away as my blood sugar dropped and my fingers stopped typing. I was certain that no one would notice. The week before the end, my mother had sent a long letter outlining how hard I'd made life for her by not vacuuming and tidying the house enough when I was a kid, but she was writing this in order to forgive me my transgressions. (This had been at the behest of her latest support-group leader who seemingly neglected to tell her the Therapy 101 step of not actually *mailing* the letter.) I lost it, I'm not proud to say, and poured a lifetime's worth of pent-up pain into the receiver. I'd been trying to keep from drowning, I told her, get through childhood and adolescence while being tugged under by her monsters and mine. I may not have been deft with a Hoover and a feather duster, but I kept everyone fed and as proud as I could make them, and that ought to count for something.

When we finally finished screaming, I was spent and there was no one to reach out to.

It was right before Christmas and all through my house, there was the detritus of the life I thought I had with this man: the Sunday *New York Times*, a shirt that still smelled like his gym sweat, a favorite book he'd lent me, kissy-face photo-booth strips from Coney Island, stockings torn off in haste. It stayed there, right where it had landed. All of it. For a long time.

Did I eat? I must have, because there's the paper bag and wax paper from the deli. Though that could have been from the day before . . . or the day before that. Diet Coke bottles all look the same once they're empty, and I meant to haul the featherlight, bulging bags of them down to the curb for recycling, but isn't that only on Tuesdays? Or is it Wednesdays? I don't want to risk getting in trouble or clattering down the stairs this late, so maybe I'll just wait and make sure. Mail: can't toss any of that out, because what if I accidentally throw away an important document and seal my financial doom? Or a piece of paper that Mumsie had written on. I might be furious at her right now, but she's not well and I have to cling on to any scrap of her I have. In fact, if I throw anything from her away—pictures, lumpy Christmas crafts, hand-scrawled cards with words that spiraled around the perimeters once she'd crowded the center (and the envelopes they came in)—it's a sign to the universe that I don't care enough about preserving her memory and I'll lose her. I'll lose it all.

It's breathtaking how quickly a home can slide into chaos, tumbling from a few scattered sheets of paper, unwashed glasses, and cast-off socks to an avalanche of mess. What would have once been an hour or two's worth of stacking, sweeping, scrubbing, and hauling suddenly became an insurmountable task. I'm so, so tired. I'll just shove it to the side, step over it. I'll deal with it tomorrow. Maybe tomorrow. Maybe tomorrow.

"Well, you know," a normal person would—and several did—say, "There are people who, for a fee, will come and alleviate this problem for you. There are even gentlemen who would come over and do such a thing for free if you let them clean your apartment naked (them, not you) and maybe yelled at them a little."

Even for free (plus yelling), there was a cost, though, mostly to my dignity. I couldn't let anyone, a professional or a live, nude volunteer, see the mortifying conditions I lived in, and I worried endlessly that some emergency would necessitate someone coming into my apartment and seeing heaps and stacks and monoliths and towers of stuff that looked like trash to a rational person's eye.

I justified to myself that my post-breakup apartment was disorganized not dirty because it was all just objects and not food. I drank only Diet Coke and recapped the bottles once I finished, and frankly, there was no possibility of cooking grime because the fridge had been manufactured before the "defrost" option was in vogue, and unless I was vigilant with a chisel and a pan of boiling water, within a week or two, the freezer compartment tended to ice over so thickly it was impossible to close the door to the whole unit. I eventually stopped storing food in there at all.

But even this didn't rouse me to call Ralph to come in and replace the damn thing. Or swap out that high-up bulb that even my loftiest chair and a teetering stack of reference books couldn't help me reach. Or adjust the radiator so I didn't fear dying of hypothermia in my bed each and every February (though I hear that's among the calmer ways to go). My cable, for which I paid a hefty sum, went on the fritz as well, and in a great show of optimism, I'd actually schedule appointments to get it fixed, and then inevitably cancel them on the day of, sick to my stomach that I'd failed, yet again, at the basic adult task of not living like a garbage monster, and completely paralyzed by the thought of another human seeing how I lived. On at least one occasion, too scared to even make the cancellation call, I'd huddled under the covers in a horror-struck ball as the doorbell rang, and rang and rang until the repairman finally gave up.

A few years and a run as a dominatrix later, I flew the nest and landed gently in Douglas's world, and oh, did I love it there. And him. And them. He traveled in a pack, flanked by Mordred, a comically grand, unnervingly nervous Irish wolfhound, and Morgane, who seemed to be constructed of one hundred percent pure, grade-A, uncut sunshine, molded into whippet form. (She peed on the rug nearly every day, but we all have our issues.)

It was easy to fall into their rhythm—an early morning, a walk, some work, some supper, some cuddles, some sleep. It was tidy and warm and lovely in their Manhattan home, if a little bit snugger than mine. (Mordred had to perform K-turns to maneuver through some parts of the slender railroad apartment.) After spending the night a dozen or so times, and parting ways with a lingering kiss on a blustery corner at 7 A.M., Douglas gave me a key to his apartment.

I thanked him profusely, I used it constantly, I couldn't return the favor.

Actually, I told myself, it wouldn't be a favor at all to subject him to that miles-deep flaw in the woman he was beginning to love. Comfort and tidiness were paramount to Douglas. He'd been born and raised in High Point, North Carolina—the furniture capital of America—by parents surprised to be once again caring for a newborn, seventeen years after the birth of their second child. His dad liked Dewar's and his mom craved as much order as she could in the face of that. Douglas learned early on that a meticulously kept home might possibly be the sticking plaster that kept the wound from bursting open from time to time. It wasn't, but you learn what you learn when you're young, and who's ever going to fault you for having a well-dusted, wood-polished, neatly appointed home?

Oh, and a church. Whereas I could barely manage the upkeep of an increasingly shabby walk-up floor-through, this new fellow of mine had almost single-handedly restored a 150-year-old Gothic, stone Episcopal church in upstate New York from a raw, unheated, barely plumbed cavern to a warm, two-bedroom home with a claw-foot tub, a granite countertop kitchen, and seating for twelve to twenty-four dinner guests in the sanctuary.

If he had a sanctuary, I had a belfry. And I wanted to keep the sanctity of it to myself as long as I could, because as God was my witness, who could love me after seeing how I lived?

Then it was my turn to flinch. After some pavement pounding, we'd found a suitably heavy-beamed, architecturally interesting apartment eleven blocks over, one block up and five flights lower than my junk-strewn hovel, with a little fenced-in area for a grill, and wide enough so that the wolfhound could maneuver without requiring rearview mirrors. We patched, painted, and emptied Douglas's apartment, lovingly rouged and gilded every surface of our (OUR!) place until it looked like Goth Barbie's Dream Home, and installed my rabbit, Claudette, in my new office behind a solidly dog-proof door.

And yet I stayed locked up in the tower, afraid to let my hair down and allow him up or me down. Daunted by the prospect of packing and tossing and hauling (oh God, all those steps—I'll be so glad to be rid of those), I'd root through and find a few obvious things to throw away (Diet Coke bottles, those can go, but did I enter the code off the cap yet? I'm so close to having enough points for another free Diet Coke . . .) and then, overwhelmed by the mass of it all, allow myself the luxury of a nap atop my clothes-strewn bed. It was just too much, too much, too much at once. I get the chocolate factory AND the Oompa Loompas AND all the fizzy lifting drink all at once? Just for being me? What's the catch? There has to be a catch.

In my fretful dreams, I'd purge and haul what was left of my belongings over to my . . . OUR new apartment only to find that he'd changed his mind or was playing an elaborate prank on me and I was suddenly homeless. Or that as soon as he had to share a bathroom and closet space with me, makeup-free, period underwear, and hair up in a messy sleep knot, he'd find me the dullest lump on the planet and wonder where I'd stashed the corpse of the corseted vamp who'd rammed her tongue down his throat that first night we met. Or maybe he expected that I'd meet him at the door every night in a freshly pressed apron with a pot roast in the oven (I can't stand pot roast) and a chilled old fashioned (those I do like) in hand for him. Oh, honey, you're home.

It got a little weird. While Douglas was nothing but patient and kind to me, Ralph was starting to tap his foot. While my lease technically was good for another six months or so, he'd promised my apartment to his nephew, who'd agreed to take over as the building's superintendent—not to mention that he was wounded by my betrayal. I'd wronged him, he said, by taking up with another man. He'd always assumed I'd be done with the boyfriends and he and I would be together. Where he got that notion, I'll never know. But it made me want to get with the packing already.

But there was a mountain of crap to get through first: clothes and papers and long-neglected art supplies and books and dishes and photos and tchotchkes and CDs and planting supplies and more papers and can't I just use this apartment as a closet for my stuff and pop by when I need something? Economically untenable, but a freaked-out girl can dream.

I've always been a lover of objects, imbuing them with meaning and emotional weight that they weren't necessarily made to bear. It's part of what drove me to be a sculptor and metalsmith in the first place: transferring the burden of feeling out of me and into materials that would not be damaged by it. It can be a good and healing thing—until you're curled up weeping in your hallway because you're afraid that if you throw away an envelope with your mother's handwriting on it, you'll have nothing to remember her by when she dies. Eight years gives a person like me an awful lot of time to accumulate things. Eight years of hauling objects up five flights to be used exclusively by me and rarely discarded. Eight years of boxing, draping, and concealing objects as needed to give the appearance that I lived like a halfway-sane human if I knew someone needed to come over. Oh, you don't want to go in the front room, it's too cold/ hot/loud for the people downstairs/full of bees, bears, and alligators. Not to mention that if you step incorrectly, you will be crushed to death by teetering knickknacks and boxes of receipts.

I finally gritted my teeth, swallowed my pride, and reached out to a friend who'd been offering help. I knew (or at least hoped) that Adair would never judge me. She's blunt and opinionated, with an unwavering sense of justice and a seemingly unlimited supply of kindness for people she feels deserve it. She is also a fellow messy person—which would seem counterintuitive to my calling her, but also meant she'd understand better than most. She walked in with an armload of packing tape and newspaper, assessed the situation, informed me that I needed to stop apologizing, and sorted out my kitchen in a matter of hours. One room down. Maybe I could get through this.

I didn't see Douglas much over the course of the next few days. I'd call him, "This is your girlfriend, Sisyphus," reporting on my progress and offering revised estimates of my move-in date. I'd finally reached out to a moving company, hitting send with a shaking finger after several days of having the e-mail in draft. And canceling the assessment meeting with the movers a few times after that. While I'd made progress, I just could not stand the notion of a stranger coming in, taking the measure of my life, and putting a price on what it would take to set it right.

I told him what I knew he needed to hear. "Baby, of course I'm not having second thoughts. You saw that I hand-carried all those cocktail glasses over and my ancient teddy bear is already in my office. No way would I leave Bombur hanging, he's been mine since I was seven! Of course we can sit down for dinner tonight. Should I . . . cook or something?"

Oh God, am I supposed to cook dinner for my live-in boyfriend? Is that what people do? Does this mean I'll have to sit down and use cutlery and napkins and make potatoes and not watch *Law & Order*? Not just gobble moo shu pork with my hands from paper plates while swigging Diet Coke straight from the bottle? Dammit. DAMMIT. He should know what he's in for, and I should give him a chance to bow out before I hand the keys back to Ralph. That's the decent thing to do. I met him at the front door.

Despite my bouts of agoraphobia, I'd been up and down the stairs a few thousand times in my eight-year residence, but the initial ascent next to Douglas may have been the steepest of all. My lungs constricted as we rose and I begged for breath at each landing. I could taste my heart. I'd been naked in front of this man in every way, but he was about to see me stripped, flayed, raw. I could see his eyes grow wide at the mountain of plastic, packed tubs I'd moved into the hallway already. No sense prolonging the pain. I shoved open the door and braced myself for his disgust, his dismissal. I led him from room to room to bear witness to the sticky, stained linoleum, the strewn clothes, the teetering paper heaps. Take it in, take it all in. This was made by the creature you were foolish enough to love and from whom you can still be free.

I dared a look at his face, searching for signs of the love draining from his eyes, replaced by pity and revulsion.

"Are you grossed out by how much of a horrible slob I am? You see why I didn't let you come over before? If you don't want to live with me, say the word. Go ahead and do it now and I'll take everything back from the apartment. Just tell me now, so we can get it over with."

He stepped forward and drew my tear-sogged, hysterical face to his shoulder, wrapping his arms around me to still me.

"I love you. Thank you for trusting me. What can I carry home to our place?"

And when the movers finally came to take everything away, the clamor and bustle lasted late into the night. When I came to give the keys to Ralph the next day and do a final walk-through, he grumbled at me. The downstairs neighbors had complained to him about all the noise we'd made on the stairs.

I made sure to stomp on every single step until I hit the landing one last time.

In my nervousness leading up to our move-in together, I'd polled married and cohabiting friends about strategies for sharing living space with a person you loved, and wanted to keep loving. I'd been terrified about constant exposure wearing away at our affection, of eight years of solitude turning me into a creature who'd startle and bolt if asked to pass the half-and-half in the morning. "Just make sure you have a door that you can put between you if need be" was the most common advice. "And three checking accounts: yours, mine, and ours."

And it worked. Enough so that ten weeks in, I tempted fate, limping in the front door on February 14, yanking off my boot, and showing Douglas his valentine in the form of a tattooed key—the front door to our apartment, in fact—with a scroll underneath emblazoned with the word "Solidarity." He'd gotten under my skin so far, made me feel so very at home, I forgot, for once, to be afraid.

IRRATIONAL FEAR #8
PICKING THINGS UP

My favorite pair of shoes lives about half a block from my house. They're not in a store window or a neighbor's item I am currently coveting. They're mine. I own them outright and I have a receipt to prove it.

I'm just afraid to go and get them.

I honestly have no excuse for this—not even some clever justification I'm making to myself. It's not that I lack the funds to bring them back into my custody or that the repair shop has inconvenient hours. I prepaid when I dropped them off, and I walk by it multiple times a week thinking, "Oh, good! I'll pick them up on my way home." I've been saying that for about six weeks now. And the longer I let it go on, the more afraid I am that when I go to pick them up, they just won't be there anymore. Or that I'll be judged for my perceived laziness and carelessness.

This is not the first time that this has happened, and unless my brain is surgically or chemically rewired, it will happen again. I'm ashamed of it and it only compounds the longer I allow it to drag on. It costs me money. If I don't go get those shoes back, I'm out a couple hundred dollars (they're really nice shoes, stylish and sturdy, which is why I bothered to get them fixed in the first place—that and the fact that I am hard-pressed to throw out useful things when they're damaged). But they're not even the most expensive object I've abandoned out of fear. The last man I dated before I met Douglas has a ring I left behind at his house, a piece of jewelry I'd bought for myself in a declaration of autonomy and independence. Perhaps it's understandable that I didn't want to see him or ask him for it in the aftermath of our split, but in the ten years hence, during which we've both married other people and established the friendship we should have just stuck to in the first place, I've been too hesitant to broach the subject.

That's actually not even the worst of it. My car was towed once—totally my fault, letting a string of tickets go unpaid for too long. At least one was for letting my inspection sticker lapse (stupid me, it was actually in my mailbox, just not on my car), and another one or two for forgetting to switch sides on street-cleaning day. Though the parking authority has since instituted online payment for tickets, if I wanted to spare myself a trip to the Finance Business Centers and the Offices of the Sheriff of Kings County, it required a physical check—which entailed finding my checkbook, locating an envelope and a stamp, and uggghhhh, a trip to the post office, because who has stamps just lying around? (Answer: most normal, useful, responsible, grown-up people who probably also know where their checkbook, Social Security card, and passport are.) The fines compounded, and one day, there my car just wasn't.

God, I felt pathetic. I hardly ever used the cursed thing, just the occasional IKEA or garden-center haul for friends. I spent hideous, wasteful, stressful hours of my life trawling neighborhood streets for legal parking. But it was *my* hideous hunk of American-made steel and I was responsible for its upkeep—or at least knowing where the heck it was.

I tracked it down to a tow yard near a decidedly unromantic ship-yard in no-man's-land Brooklyn. They only accepted cash, along-side a receipt from the marshal's office saying my original fine and all penalty fees had been paid in full. And it was a lot of cash—way more than my ATM would allow me to withdraw in a single day, or even two. It was either rip the Band-Aid off, remove the whole sum at once, find a way to schlepp out and pay the ransom for my Tau-rus's release—which would have been the sane, fiscally sound, and adult thing to do or . . . OR I could take the cash out in dribs and drabs and allow the storage fees to mount.

Oh yeah—the sprinkle of sugar in the gas tank here: the facility charged an additional ten dollars a day for the first three days and fifteen a day after that for the burden of housing deadbeats' cars. And still, something stopped me.

I was mortified; that was definitely part of it. That I'd let things get this bad—the original fines and the mounting penalties. I harbored fantasies of wobbling timidly toward an ornate, filigreed gate, possibly over a moat filled with junkyard dragons, hungry for the blood of debtors, and hearing my name proclaimed over a boom-ing loudspeaker: "Miss Kinsman, we'd been wondering when you would show your face." After standing on tiptoe to hand the fistful of hundreds over the high counter to a sneering official, likely in a curled wig and ornate robe, I'd be led past a phalanx of workers who'd all come out to see what kind of sorry excuse for a human would be so irresponsible, out to the center of a tumbleweed-strewn lot that housed my car and only my car. "Phew!" they'd say. "We can finally go home to our families now."

This did not happen. I handed over my forms and a depressingly thick envelope of bills to a completely disinterested woman behind a counter in a wood-paneled trailer, wearing a polo shirt and watching her stories on a portable TV. My car was one of hundreds, if not thousands, of cars jammed into the chain-link-fenced lot out by the docks. Some had clearly been abandoned for good, if the layers of seagull droppings were any indication of their owners' commitment to reclamation. New cars were being towed in to take the place of those belonging to grim-faced owners who forked over the cash and turned their keys. Some were clunkers, others shiny, bright, and pricey. Seriously, dude, there's your Benz. You don't have the time and cash to come claim it? Then again, I had both those things and still it took me weeks to come get my car.

Maybe those other owners were like me—afraid of the judgment that earned interest by the day, making it harder and harder to come and claim what's theirs. Perhaps it's the fear that comes and bloodies your skin if you've ever been broke and hopeless. Even if you claw your way out, earn enough money to form a thick suit of armor, being forced to spend any of it leaves you feeling like the wound has been stripped open again. Maybe they, too, had been raised to feel like correction and punishment are the signs of a loving deity and to pay penance—even to a random and seemingly godless tow yard—was somehow deserved and even a little divine. I'll never know. I fired up the engine and drove the hell out of there and parked oh-so-carefully.

Douglas had an aging, faithful Jeep that through the transitive powers of cohabitation and Geico policies effectively became mine as well. My Taurus, nicknamed Russell, increasingly unreliable on the four-hour highway trip between Brooklyn and the church, was sent to live out the remainder of his days upstate to be used for grocery jaunts or possibly donation to a local charity. But as was his wont, one day there he wasn't. I'd left him parked in front of the church a couple of weeks before, and there must have been snowfall. There are laws about such things in towns where plowing is paramount, but I hadn't been in a position to do anything about it. Still, the town where the church is doesn't even have its own police force, let alone a squad of marshals tasked with augmenting the town's revenue with fines from parking violations. I called the village hall during one of the few hours a week it was open and was referred to the county department that deals with that kind of thing. They sort of maybe recalled having processed it, but they'd have to check and get back to me.

No one ever did. And when it came out a year or so later that the woman in charge of official village matters—like, say, collecting local taxes and the towing of cars—had been fired for misappropriation of funds and giving herself unauthorized annual raises, I let myself off the hook a little. Just a little. For once, my fear and the resultant negligence weren't at fault for something and that made me feel if not good, just a little less terrible about myself. My car hadn't disappeared because of my crippling anxiety! How original!

And if that makes me sound pathetic, so be it. Anxiety *can* be a crippling beast, so try to hobble a mile in my shoes.

But you'll have to pick them up, first.

CHAPTER TEN

On Money and Futons

I was on my way into the city to get fired when a man I'd never met jumped in front of the L-train and ended his life. This method of dispatch happens far more often than most people know, but if your ears are open to it, you can figure out what's gone down. "Police investigation," they often tell people stranded on increasingly crowded platforms up and down the line. Officially a "12–9" in departmental code. If a motorman hits and kills someone, they are required to take three days off from work. Many come back, some take longer, and some never return.

This time, the conductor ditched the lingo, so we all knew what was up, cawing over the PA system: "Listen, next station says this is gonna take a while to clean up, so you might as well walk over to the J/M/Z train at Marcy Avenue. Good luck."

While my skin had certainly thickened in the two years I'd lived in New York City at this point, it was nowhere near its current rhinolike density. The words of my fellow frustrated commuters that day bugged me. "Asshole! Why's his last move on earth gotta be screwing the rest of us over like this?" "Jerk like that probably pulled selfish shit like this all the time. Good riddance."

I joined the swarm up the stairs to street level. Blood pounding in my skull to the cadence of my steps, I marched across the neighborhood to the train that would haul me across the river to my own doom. And with every thud, I blamed him less. Maybe his boss had called him to a mysterious outside-the-office meeting, too, and he knew it was the end of the road for him. Only one more step to take.

This job had saved me from a constantly growling stomach, eviction, constant sickness from living in an illegal, mostly unheated loft where I breathed in sawdust kicked up by my sculptor roommate. I inhaled contempt from the socialist one, who scorned me for owning a television (that she often borrowed), and goodness knows what from the homeless man our other roommate had met by the docks and was now boning. I'd sent out tens, dozens, scores of résumés after fleeing my previous job and had a few nibbles here and there, some freelance, but not enough to keep my landlord from banging on the door in search of his $500 cash each month when I was late.

I'd quit my last position without much of a plan in place, other than to make the panic stop. It's not as if I'd left an especially lucrative, lucky opportunity behind, but it did come with insurance and $442.30 a week before taxes, which was 442.3 times more than I was making now. It was also a damn sight more than the no-benefits minimum-wage jobs I'd stacked up for the previous year and a half. I'd taken the job as the office manager of a small graphic design firm in part because I was too afraid to apply for—and be rejected from—any actual design positions. It was art-adjacent, I told myself, and harbored fantasies that the boss would somehow sniff out my untapped potential as I filed, billed, and set up the company website and e-mail (it was the midnineties and I felt mildly godly for possessing that level of tech savvy). Maybe he'd take a chance on this scrappy kid and let me sub in while one of the real designers was on vacation. Then he'd see. Then they'd all see.

And if nothing else, being in close proximity to a pilot light of creative inspiration would fuel my creative brain. I'd burst free from the dull but restful bonds of my mindless office toil and spend my evenings, weekends, and early mornings making paintings and collages and possibly a redux of my groundbreaking bird-related performance art, too.

None of that happened, and if I did lift an eyelid before my morning alarm, it was because I'd been jolted awake by a stress nightmare or a creak that sounded suspiciously like someone trying to break into my bedroom. My "easy" job turned out to be unexpectedly challenging work made infinitely worse by a boss who couldn't keep his temper in check, his fingers from the company till, or his soft, meaty paws off the all-female staff.

But it's not as if you can screen for those sorts of things in an interview, especially in a boss.

"Do you offer both dental and vision, and by the way, have any of your senior employees had to take several months away from the workforce after leaving your company because you emotionally abused them so badly they were unable to work for a while?"

"Where do you see the company in six months? Do you see it backing its youngest, most poorly paid employee against the break room sink and sticking its tongue down her throat and traumatizing her so badly she quits the next day via answering machine and moves back home to Japan?"

"Is there room for advancement in the company? Say, moving on from receiving the insurance a longtime employee relies on to manage her chronic liver condition to being told she should piggyback on her husband's because it's just so expensive for the firm to have to pay all these employees' benefits that are part of their basic compensation packages?"

"What are the expected work hours? If an employee arrives at her appointed time of eight forty-five A.M., will she be able to tell if the employer is already in the office just from the way the air feels and immediately feel like vomiting on her shoes? Additionally, will the employee be allowed to take her lunch break after three P.M., at which point she can afford the half-price soup from the deli nearby *and* they set out the big, stale breakfast rolls and are happy to let her have one of them instead of crackers and she can have her one decent meal of the day?"

"If the owner's wife starts working at the company as well, will she also be in a position to bring each employee into her office to tell them, as a courtesy from a seasoned professional and avid practitioner of yoga, what they're lacking as workers and as human beings?"

"Is the supply closet large enough to accommodate more than two or three sobbing employees at a time?"

"What is the average number of weeks or months after quitting it takes an employee of your company to stop waking up hyperventilating, flinching when the phone rings, or avoiding the block where the office is?"

"How many times will the average employee of your firm regret having resigned, even if she is unable to find work, has to hide from the landlord, can't afford heat, and finds it nearly impossible to leave her house, bedroom, or bed for several months?"

The answer to that last one is zero. Zero times.

It would have been easy to mistake me for lazy right then. Not speaking, not waking, not doing, not making—just breathing, and badly at that. I'd been in constant motion for a year and a half since moving to New York City, scrambling from apartment to apartment, job to job, clawing after every cent I could to prove I was worthy of living in this sharp-edged place—or anywhere for that matter. And I was failing miserably.

If I wasn't working and earning, then what was the point of my existing at all? That value system had been twisted into my genetic makeup. Mumsie's siblings were a priest, social worker, nurse, and teacher. She herself had taught English, then religious education before she became unable to. My mother and her brothers and sisters were not allowed time away from school in the summer or the freedom to simply be kids. As the sons and daughters of first-generation Americans, Catholic to the core, they had to be bettering themselves and the world around them or else. Else what, I'm not sure. Perhaps that they'd be told they could not stay. This land is our land, but not your land.

Her father had been made to feel that way—not all the hard work in the world, not a bachelor's or master's degree or a job engineering parts for *Air Force One* could stop people from hurling the word "WOP" at the poor little shoeless boy whose mother took in washing and never learned much English. He refused to eat garlic because he didn't want to "smell Italian." His immigrant father-in-law built a successful fruit importing business from the ground up, and still, he'd only ever be "Banana Tony" to the people in that small Pennsylvania town.

Pup's parents worked themselves to the bone, his father nearly bleeding to death on a customer's icy front porch, artery nicked on a broken bottle along his milk run. They still almost lost the house a few times, and he cried when he couldn't spare the fifty cents for his son to go bowling with his friends. So if all this work doesn't get you where you need to feel safe, worthy, and welcome, what's the point? Unless you somehow win the lottery (though who would waste their money on that?) or woo a billionaire into wedded bliss, you don't get to decide. You just keep doing.

And sometimes the doing wasn't good enough. I'd hustled my way through school, chasing every opportunity and accolade in an effort to prove myself worthy to colleges—and, frankly, to get the hell out of my increasingly unstable house. But the tone of disgust in Grandfather Ribando's voice on the Sunday call in which he was told that I'd opted for art school made me feel like a soot-faced, barefoot urchin tugging at the hem of the town swell's overcoat. I wasn't actually asking him for anything—not even his approval— but in his eyes, declaring my intent to make a life in the arts was essentially stepping up to the world with my hand out.

I could have won the Olympic downhill sloth championship with my efforts that winter after quitting my job. All I did was sleep. It was free, for one thing, and the less I moved, the less I needed to eat and buy and expose my skin to the freezing air. I was certain my grandpa Kinsman, up before dawn to saddle the horse that pulled his dairy truck, or my grandfather Ribando, learning fundamental cobbling techniques so he wouldn't have to stumble to school bare-foot, would be extremely proud of their granddaughter, hunched all day and night under her filthy polyester comforter in an unheated Brooklyn warehouse because she was too damned scared that some-one might yell at her again or tell her she wasn't good enough. .

And then the sun came out. Literally: the sun came out one day in early April and it was suddenly warm and I could crawl out of my bed and shower for more than ten seconds without fear that my skin was going to fall off in frosty chunks. I sent out résumés left and right, so emboldened by my desperation that I was throwing my hat in the ring for actual design jobs, in addition to office support staff.

The fear that had debilitated me, pinned me to my reeking,

lumpy futon for all those months, was what finally pushed me forward. Be afraid of living on the street, hunger, assault, a deep-lung cough you can't afford to treat. Being afraid of the word "no" and having your pride wounded isn't a luxury you can afford.

I got my dream job—an entry-level design position at an online city guide that paid about 80 percent more than what I'd been making at the last gig, working under a supervisor who only made me cry once. That came about when he must have overheard me whispering on the phone to a friend that payroll was late with my first check and I'd stayed at the office until after dark, and I didn't have enough money for both dinner and subway fare, so could I maybe walk downtown, take the free ferry to Staten Island, and crash at her house that night? Robert showed up at my desk with twenty-five dollars and a story about how if you work past a certain hour, you'd get money for a car home. I held my tears back until he walked away, since he'd gone to such an effort to let me keep my dignity. A check showed up from payroll the next day.

And with that first paycheck, I fulfilled a small pact I'd made with myself in the empty-gutted worst of it. Not a new dress or a trip or a spa visit; I pushed a cart through the grocery store and bought what I wanted, even allowing myself name-brand items if they weren't outrageous. My arms were sore for days from lugging it all home. I didn't mind a bit.

It's astonishing how much more you can accomplish when you're warm, safe, and fed—and how hungry you are to hold on to that. I soared under Robert's guidance, so grateful he'd picked my portfolio out of the pile, been willing to take a chance on a fairly untested designer (which might have been a matter of budget restraints, but still), and I was not about to let him worry that he'd misplaced his faith. I knew I might be a little bit behind—metalsmithing and web design only have so much overlap—so I rushed to catch up, leaving the office last every night and copying files onto clunky Zip disks to fuss over at home until the wee, small hours. I made it in by at least the crack of ten most mornings and skipped lunch to make up for it.

Anything I hadn't been taught to do correctly, I figured out my own way to execute—interestingly enough that no one would notice I was covering up my shortcomings. I've used this strategy countless times throughout my career. Then, I didn't know how to use Adobe Illustrator or Flash, so I figured out how to make cheeky little drawings in Photoshop, which I'd taught myself after hours at the graphic design firm, and turn them into animated gifs. Later on, as a freelance webmaster, I stitched together bits of code I scraped from website source files and poked at them until they seemed to talk properly to the SQL databases I'd somehow managed to install. (I'm still gob-smacked that I managed to pull that one off, but when they'd asked if I knew how to program, I just said yes.)

And when I got hired to write about food for CNN, I spent the first two years huddled at my desk waiting for someone to figure out that I wasn't a real reporter, and send security to toss me out onto Columbus Circle. Possibly while Anderson Cooper flipped me the bird. I fake it until I give the rough appearance of making it—and, to be fair to myself, do a crap-ton of work along the way—bracing for the reveal all the while.

Back then at the city guide, Robert seemed to believe in me—but he didn't actually have a design background, so he wasn't going to find me out. And the interim editor in chief—she was just trying to keep the ship afloat, and besides, I was a friend of her boyfriend. She was just giving me a pass until the real boss showed up. It was just a matter of time, I told myself.

When he did arrive, it was in the form of a quick-witted, prema-

turely silver-haired man named Sean, with a two-decade publish-
ing track record and a well-honed bullshit sensor. He took his time,
settled in, observed, tweaked, shuffled the editorial staff, shaking
out what wasn't solidly locked down. And then he fixed his gaze on
the production team. It was just two of us by that point. Robert had
set sail for more lucrative seas at a financial website, hiring Ali in
his stead. We'd formed as a tight crew quickly, churning out what
was asked, and even a little bit more—but still my gut lurched when
Sean asked us both to meet him outside the office in a couple of
days.

"What do you think he wants?" "I mean, he can't fire us both
because then there wouldn't be anyone to produce the website,
right?" "We can both kinda do each other's jobs—maybe he'll make
us pick which one is staying?" "Should we get another drink?" "Oh,
hell yeah. Or . . . maybe I shouldn't spend any money until I know
for sure."

Paranoia loves a partner, and that conversation Tilt-A-Whirled
through my skull as I paced on the elevated platform. These days, I'd
have lobbed half a dozen "On my way!" "Sorry!" "Almost there!"
texts across the water, but I was at least a year out from buying my
first Nokia. Ali was probably already there, always on time. They
were getting chummy. She was making her case for herself—no, for
both of us. She'd never do that to me. I scrabbled down in my bag
for change and got in line for the pay phone. Four-one-one first. Yes,
I'll accept the charge to be connected. Could you please tell them
I'm on my way? Thank you.

I crash-landed at their restaurant table, a good forty-five minutes
late and babbling out apologies: train delay, suicide, sorry. Ali looked
relaxed, sitting back with a glass of wine, and kicked me lightly
under the table. Oh God.

Sean smiled. Told me to get a glass of wine if I wanted one, but he himself didn't drink. To cushion the blow, I knew it. I sat stiffly until Sean proposed a toast: "To a really great team!"

I couldn't take it anymore. "You're not . . . firing us?"

He stared at me for a full two seconds before bursting into laughter. "Who did this to you? You really think this is how it works? If you were getting fired, it would be behind closed doors in the office with someone from HR present. And you'd get a bunch of warnings first. I'm taking you two out because you've been impressing the hell out of me and I wanted to say thank you."

In my (minor) defense, I'll note that a few years down the line at another job, I was indeed part of a catered mass layoff, but his message was received. I unclenched a little bit, tried to relax—or at least what passes for that in my body and brain.

Sean told me I could write—scratch that, *should* write in addition to my design duties. He and the music editor, Lissa, got a kick out of the e-mails I wrote to the editorial team and seemed to appreciate my taste in music, books, and food, and they put me in the semiregular rotation of reviewers. I said yes, grateful and terrified that I'd let them down.

And for the next nine years, I bobbed along in a way that passed as successful. Became a damn decent designer who took jobs at lad mags like *Maxim* and *FHM* and brands with a sense of humor. I slipped writing in when editorial and agency teams were short-staffed or under the gun, and felt lucky for the chance each time, even if no one would ever know it was my words.

I worked hard. If you want to distract someone—even yourself—you don't hide. Not when you're anxious and afraid of being unmasked as a fraud. You grab the sparkliest baton and costume you can and hope they blind everyone to your shortcomings. Leave them dazzled and breathless, then go home, strip down, and calculate if you've earned your keep that day. If not, then no rest for you; work more until you drop from exhaustion. In the morning, your bank is back down to zero and you have to fill it up again.

Other people are allowed to rest, but not me, never me. Not the anxious one. They're enough, just by the fact of their existence. They can take breaks, go on vacation, have a life, interest, hobbies, friends that don't revolve around what they do for a living, but not when you're Mumsie's daughter, her father's granddaughter. Let your limbs still for a second and you'll sink, taking everything and everyone with you.

I was making a thoroughly respectable living as a freelance copywriter at a Madison Avenue advertising agency, writing website copy, banner ads, and tag lines for cheap tequilas and facial cleansers, when the offer came in via a friend who knew I loved food. It was temporary—a summer-long gig as the grilling editor for AOL, and the agency offered to take me back on full-time at the end of it. Six months into marriage with Douglas and feeling more stable than ever before, I took the leap, landed firmly, and ran.

The food editor left in my first few weeks, and I got her job, and then the senior editor was laid off, so I took over her job, too, and I worked and worked and worked and worked to make up for the fact that I'd gotten it all by accident. And so they didn't realize that I wasn't supposed to be there.

I guess I fooled them all. I then got a job creating a food site for CNN and I spent the first few years terrified that my colleagues would figure out that I wasn't a journalist. That I was just writing this cute little food blog while they were doing the work that actually meant something. So I worked and worked and worked until I learned from them how to be a journalist, too. I won awards, respect, my place at the table.

And I was still terrified.

Here's the thing: the higher up you climb, the harder it is to hide. When you screw up in the big gig—or someone thinks you did—it's in high definition, broadcast on millions of TVs and computer monitors across the globe. And people won't hesitate to tell you all about it.

You write an article about witnessing a pig slaughter (and enjoying the ham afterward), pick a Twitter fight with Anthony Bourdain (we made up later), or suggest that Paula Deen consider giving credit to the African American cooks whose recipes her success is based on (still waiting for that), you have to expect blowback. Maybe even death threats. It means people are paying attention and taking what you say seriously. It means I am doing my job. Once I took the leap and someone decided to pay me to be a full-time writer and editor, the very worst thing I could do was to be afraid of having a strong opinion. Do your homework, back it up with facts when you can, and you're bulletproof—that was my game.

That doesn't mean you don't sob like a baby when a producer for *The Daily Show* takes a screen-grab of your face during a TV segment about solo dining, tweets it out with a caption about it being a "cry for help," and it goes viral, complete with commentary about how of course you eat alone all the time, what with you being so ugly.

It doesn't mean that when a hundred thoughtful comments pour in over an article you wrote, you won't fixate on the one that called you a banal writer, reading it over and over again until you could recite it in your sleep. (That person knows . . . they KNOW and they're the one who sees the truth.)

And it definitely doesn't mean that you don't come close to vomiting each time you send a story—big or small—to your editor, certain that this is going to be the one that exposes you to the world for the fraud you really are.

From there I spiral. Then I sink.

All hell breaks loose in my head, but no one can know. It doesn't even have to be brought on by anything in particular. My terror has a hair trigger and it can be set off by a long pause from my boss, a side glance from a colleague, a particularly lengthy silence after an e-mail—something that means absolutely nothing real, but which I take to spell my doom. My brain fills the blanks with all the terrible things it imagines the other person must be thinking, all the while whispering to me that this will just cushion the blow when it finally lands. This is bad work. You have been doing bad work for a while. You were only hired because someone felt sorry for you. But that's come to an end. They've found out what an unqualified, talent-free, hideous human you truly are and this will be their excuse to finally get rid of you. You'll be fired. Word will spread about why and everyone will agree. You'll be unhirable. You'll lose your home. You'll be hungry. You'll be alone. It was only a matter of time before you're back on the futon.

I found my voice when I started writing about food. It had sustained me in all the usual ways, and maybe some that weren't. In the thick of my mother's illness—the physical parts at least—I took to cooking our family dinner. Especially after Nan was off at college and it was just the three of us, if she was bedridden for a spell after surgery, I'd come home from play rehearsal, yearbook meetings, cheerleading practice and cobble together the most nourishing meals I could muster from the binder-spined *Betty Crocker Cookbook* that had been living in our kitchen since the dawn of time. When Pup got home from work, we made three plates and woke Mumsie to hunker around her bed, bolstering our family bond with ketchup-clotted meat loaf, clunkily breaded pork chops, and every soup-can casserole on God's green earth.

On weekends, when she was sleeping or in group prayer, Pup and I prowled the greater Cincinnati area in search of flavors other than our own, exploring the world in a safe radius from her if she needed us to come home quickly. When he took me to Baltimore to visit the college I ended up attending, he built in time for a meal at Tony Cheng's—a then-famous Szechuan place where I scorched my throat on kung pao squid for the first time, but far from the last. On the drive from Kentucky to Maryland with my clothes, posters, tapes, and art supplies in tow, we fortified ourselves with patty melts at truck stops and shared a final, teary (me, not him) meal at a greasy spoon diner that reminded him of his own undergrad years. He stuffed a few twenties in my fist and drove back home.

Eating is one of the very few things that everyone on earth must do to remain alive, and it's as vibrant as language. Transcends it, often. When that first grilling-editor job dropped into my lap, my purpose was tethered to it—a note tied to a rock, lobbed through my front window. I had to heed it.

For the first time in my career, I put my trembling, bitten skin in the game. I'd always worked hard, long, maniacally to justify my worth and keep the wolves from the door, but it was always at a remove, unbylined, for a brand, laminated in protective irony so the damns I gave wouldn't easily dent. But now, speak or forever hunger for your piece of the pie.

I'd learned how to research and report bulletproof stories, and when I began sneaking a small taste of first person into my food writing, readers didn't seem to spit it out. Maybe I'd earned it, and maybe they liked it. I kept on going. It was for context, I told myself, and just for seasoning. But that's what people latched on to—even asked for more.

What I found out pretty quickly was that if you can find this common ground of pleasure with people, you can also start to talk a little bit about the pain. Because we all use a certain amount of sugar to balance the sour. You have to be able to get up and be a human being in the world on any given day, and you have to feed yourself to keep doing that.

My mother is ill—oh, I remember this goulash she used to make when she wasn't well. She's been hospitalized again—hey, look at this great chicken soup recipe I made for my dad. September 11th happened—here are the nachos I ate to numb myself.

I raised the flame. It finally came to a boil. My colleague Ann ran the Geek Out! blog at CNN. It covered fandom and identity, and she asked if I'd write an essay about being a teenage Goth. Without allowing myself a moment to panic, I vomited out several decades' worth of pent-up angst—with enough remove and humor to poke fun at myself, and finally some compassion for that weird little bat I'd been—complete with a picture of my seventeen-year-old spike-haired self in black lipstick and a dog collar. Maybe it would be of use to someone, I thought. I hit send.

When my colleagues at CNN Living were shorthanded during a month themed around the topic of beauty, I volunteered to write about how I'd finally come to not mind my big nose so much, and maybe even like it a little. It's not as if I could hide it, what with it being as plain as the . . . you know. I gave Elle her first cameo—the day she had me curled into a ball on a hotel room carpet during a class trip, flicking and grabbing my nose and telling me how ugly I was and would never be loved. I'd let her whisper my story to me for such a long time, even years after I'd heard her voice for the last time. I wrested the pen. I wrote me down.

Send. Boom.

A month and a half later, on Mother's Day weekend, CNN ran

my essay about knowing I'd never have or want children. Sixteen thousand likes, shares, comments—thank you for putting words to the thing I'd always felt, always had to justify.

One lone commenter wrote in to say that I'd failed in my existence as a woman. I addressed my feelings on that on live television. I'd never been less terrified.

But these were empirical things about me. Look at my face, my high-school-yearbook photos, the lack of tiny shoes and tuition bills in my home, and you can gather these facts. It felt like a lie of omission to be publicly praised for my honesty, yet leave out the thing I kept hidden in plain sight. So I wrote about depression. My depression. Boom.

The day two years prior when the tax bill showed up was nearly my last on earth. It was my fault entirely, this piece of paper with the precise tally of my failure as an adult human being: $24,832.62 worth of uselessness on my part. Would have been a lot less had I actually dealt with the issue in the several years I'd been receiving increasingly thick and dire IRS envelopes, but I didn't, and there it was.

Thinking back on it now, some years removed from that afternoon, is like running a finger over a deep scrape that's only just beginning to scab over. It's toughened just a little—enough so my meat, nerves, and blood are less exposed to the elements—but all it takes for me to reel back to the full body shock, sweat drench, and short circuit of those dire hours is a vaguely official-looking envelope dropped through the front door slot, or worse, a slip of paper informing me that there's a registered letter awaiting me at the post office. I'm in purgatory until I can sprint there, with a government-issued ID.

Holy hell, do I hate the mail.

But I, personally, Katherine Kinsman, neglected to pay my 2004 taxes. I could have sworn I did. In my mind's eye, I can see myself gathering up receipts, combing through my online credit-card statements, slaving over Turbo Tax, and hitting the send button and/or printing the whole mess out, scribbling a check I hoped to heaven would clear, and sprinting to stand in line for a premidnight postmark on that IRS-bound envelope. I may have indeed engaged in large chunks of those activities, but apparently not enough to actually count.

The day the "we're deadly serious and if we don't hear from you, we'll drain your bank account, shame you to your neighbors, and possibly even sell your organs for scrap" letter came, the panic metastasized in my chest and knocked me down onto my bed. There was absolutely no getting around the fact that this was my fault, with compounded interest, and now it was time for me to pay up for my failures as a human. As an adult. As a wife—oh, hell. We'd only just exhaled from a white-knuckle year and a half in which Douglas had finally broken free from his chaotic, addict business partner and the real estate market had tanked. We'd been on lockdown, tallying every cent (whither those carefree days of chucking whatever I wanted into the grocery basket), begging for grace from our kindhearted landlord, and doing our best to save face with our friends and families. Why burden them with our worries? But can we please draw names this Christmas instead of buying presents for everyone? Maybe just this once? We've both just been so . . . busy. That part wasn't a lie.

Eventually the market turned. We both got new jobs and began to fill the hole of debt we'd dug ourselves into. Back out one night at our favorite neighborhood restaurant—hey, you two! Haven't seen you for what, it seems like at least a year. Thought we'd lost you.

Now I'd dragged us back down into the pit, under the dirt, choking on it. Maybe . . . the thought shot from my heart to my throat . . . maybe this is where I belong. Let Douglas go free, climb up and out away from me, and he can see the sun again, enjoy the fruits of his labor. Maybe that was the kindest thing I could do. He'd never leave me of his own accord. "Solidarity, baby!" had been our rallying cry since that very first online message five years before, and I'd stuck by his side while we lived as close to the bone as we could.

I'll free him, I thought. He'll thank me one day, see it was all for the best.

Sorry, my darling—I cannot leave things neatly, but I can go with love. I stepped outside of myself and watched as Douglas came home, found me curled up in our dark bedroom with the IRS letter next to me. I wasn't ready yet, so I choked down dinner while he told me he'd call his accountant first thing in the morning. "I'm so, so sorry," I said over and over so he'd have extra when he needed it. We went to bed and I waited for his breathing to slow. I kissed his head, laid my hand on the whippet's chest, and felt her heart beat.

It couldn't be pills. That would be a defeat. I'd never quite had the guts to ask Pup exactly what had happened all those years back when Mumsie crashed, but I had my suspicions. And moreover, pills were what she had been made of ever since that moment.

Not the closet, not a razor, not anything extra that Douglas would have to clean up. He loves this home and he doesn't need it haunted. What, then?

A subway line runs under our building. The rumbling unnerved me for the first few months, clinking the dishes and the liquor bottles at regular intervals. I grew up close enough to a fault line that I mistook it for minor earthquakes before I mostly stopped noticing it, but as I lay in bed that night, it barreled right through me. I crept downstairs to get closer. At that hour, the F-train comes every twenty minutes. Rush hour starts at roughly six fifteen. It takes an hour to get things cleared—maybe longer to assemble an iron-stomached team in the middle of the night. If I'd learned anything from that man who'd ended his suffering under the L-train all those years ago, it's that you incur an awful lot of rotten karma if you keep your fellow citizens from getting to work. If I didn't want that tacked on to my mounting tab, I'd have to leave soon. Okay . . . now. Okay . . . now. Don't make it worse than you already have.

I stayed alive twenty minutes at a time that night, exhausting myself with the mental math and drinking in the image of my sleeping husband until I finally lay down next to him. Once the danger had passed, I was too spent to be especially useful, but I hauled myself to work out of sheer gratitude. Nothing worse could happen to me than I'd planned to do to myself.

Screw shame. Screw fear. Screw all the voices in my head telling me to be quiet, ashamed, and careful. Look where that had gotten me. What more did I have to lose?

In a series of essays and on-screen interviews, I came out to CNN's audience of millions—not to mention my bosses, colleagues, future employers, friends, and family—as mentally ill. First as having depression. Then as suffering from occasionally crippling anxiety and panic. Each time I hit send, I collapsed to the floor, emptied, terrified, certain that I'd blown my life up for good this time. Each time I switched on the beacon—I'm here, I'm flawed, I'm scared, I'm not ashamed—a thousand, two, ten, twenty blinked back in the darkness. I'm here, too. We're not alone. Let's help each other find the way.

You can get paid for all kinds of things. Money is money. The same dollars earned by sweeping floors, selling weed, making widgets, chasing debts, drawing blood, driving subways, defending crooks, pouring drinks, shining shoes, curing coughs, or landing planes can all be exchanged for the same roll of toilet paper. (Though your desired number of plies and intricacies of quilting may vary.)

But I think a lot of us who suffer from anxiety feel like we were born with an extra, invisible row on our balance sheet—where the work we do only counts under certain conditions. For some, their little internal accountant is tallying up fame, titles, accolades, awards, thank-yous, approving words from a parent, envy by a long-time rival, things to rub in the face of a bully, teacher, or boss who said they'd never amount to much.

Mine compulsively counts up acts of good. Nowadays I get called brave for my writings, speeches, and TV appearances on some scary, taboo topics, and made myself into a megaphone for people suffering from mental illness, but who don't have the luxury of speaking out. But honestly, I don't know any other way to be.

As an editor, I ask writers, "What's the story only you can tell?" I advise them to make their mark that way and trust the money to follow. As a boss, I find what shines brightest inside each member of my team, even if they can't see it, and help them to own it. For my colleagues and friends, I like to make connections. My mantra there: I'll get you laid and paid—just not for the same thing. For an employer, I'll work myself to the bone out of gratitude that they took the chance and fear they'll find they made the wrong choice.

It might not be the healthiest way to make a living, but it's the bed I made, and I'm going to lie in it, grateful every day that it's not a lumpy damn futon.

IRRATIONAL FEAR #9
DRIVING

The first time I ever drove myself to school, I crashed into my neighbor's BMW. Maybe I tapped it. Okay, I don't even know if I made contact, but I was turning the car around in the cul-de-sac, running late as usual, and I just didn't know how things were supposed to feel. I'd passed my driving test just the day before (and gotten a mustachioed mouth kiss from the pervy driver's-ed teacher—apparently a rite of passage with him), but hadn't spent much time navigating Mumsie's car, which presented its own challenges. For one, the "Slutmobile" had a bed instead of a passenger's seat because it hurt her too much to sit up for very long. (No need for a rockin', windowless van for this teen virgin queen—howzabout turning this Dodge Lancer into a sweet hump rocket with a makeshift mattress that runs from front to back, and a bitchin' hand brake for when the action gets a little too fast?) Great for comedy's sake or transporting ladders, brooms, or lawn Santas, but less so for newly licensed drivers who'd spent the bulk of their practice hours in standard cars with a copilot patiently indicating the whereabouts of curbs, pedestrians, outdoor cats, and long-haul trucks bearing down upon you on the local freeway. And parked cars. They zoom up out of nowhere, and if you're just becoming attuned to ascertaining your place in space by looking at side mirrors, they can come as a shock.

What I think actually happened is that I saw the car, braked hard, and mistook the jolt for a crash. Mortified, I threw the Slutmobile in park and felt my breakfast burning its way back up my throat as I got out and inspected the BMW's bumper for what I assumed would be complete annihilation. So far as I could tell, there was a barely perceptible scratch of indeterminate vintage, but with these fancy cars, who knew? I climbed back in and spent the rest of the school day distracted, dizzy with fear, convinced I'd come home to irate neighbors, their lawyers, furious parents, a flashing sheriff's car, and a payment plan that stretched somewhere into the twenty-second century.

And I've spent the rest of my driving years expecting a similar fate. After college, I've mostly lived in cities where my radius was small and walkable or broad and subway accessible, and that's somewhat by design. A car was a necessary evil in grad school; I'd been fibbed to by a second-year student who'd claimed the house was a bikable distance from campus, yet somehow neglected to mention the annual four-foot snow dumps that made the driveway—let alone the roads—impassable without four-wheel drive and hardcore tires. I drove only as needed, learned to swerve for deer, bears, and tipsy freshmen as well as the subtle art of convincing other people to take the wheel of my car even when I was sober.

It's not even the potential crashing so much as it is the logistics that bother me. When I get there, will I be able to find legal parking? What if I don't and I get towed? What if I miss my exit and I get turned around and suddenly I'm in the middle of a lightless swamp, slowly sinking in quicksand? What if I'm in the left lane and an aggressive driver is bearing down and I can't get over and he thinks poorly of me and I'm confirming every dumb stereotype he has about female drivers and okay he passed me and . . . gross, is that a scrotum on his bumper? What is that weird smoky smell, is my engine on fire? Is that siren part of the song, or am I being pulled over for something I was unaware I was doing? How did I get here—I think I must have blacked out for this past hundred feet. Did I hit a cow or blow a stop sign? Maybe I should pull over . . . but is that the turn to that parking lot? Will it be too hard to pull back into traffic if I stop here? I'll keep going . . . I'll keep going.

And yes, it's the crashing, too. I live in gut-wrenching terror of accidentally causing physical harm to another person. When I was very little, I rushed out in the street in front of a neighbor's car, and he screeched to a halt just in time. While he was admittedly going much too quickly on a dead-end street riddled with kids, there's no way he could have anticipated that I'd dash out in front of him. I heard later that he went home and threw up from the shock, and I felt intensely guilty for having put him in that awful emotional place.

Various bridge authorities around the country have services that cater to gephyrophobics, offering a driver for the span so the sufferer can get where they need to go without passing out or swerving off into the water. Depending on where you live, that may or may not be an issue, but there are surely destinations that require you making left-hand turns in your life. A friend and neighbor of my aunt suffered from such an intense fear of making left-hand turns that she'd have to pad her arrival time to accommodate a right-hand-only route. Others, who may have lost a loved one in an accident, survived or caused one themselves, witnessed a collision, are simply too angst-ridden to drive. Or just, like me, they may dread it for no rational reason, just a deep dread of crashing into the "maybe" that may dart from out of nowhere.

I'd love to get a bunch of us together to talk about it, but we'd have to hire a bus. And a driver.

IRRATIONAL FEAR #10

BEING DRIVEN

When I was in high school, Pup left for a business trip and it fell to me to drive him to the airport. He traveled a fair amount for his job at his chemical company, and Mumsie was always uneasy the whole time he was out of town. She tried to minimize the time they were apart, both, I assume, because they actually like each other and because she looks to him for her own calm and stability. She also spends a lot of time worrying on others' behalf (a behavior I have absorbed like a high-tech, moisture-wicking emotional sponge), and though I had been driving for at least a year at that point, she had concerns over my navigating the twenty-minute trip from our home to the greater Cincinnati International Airport. I had concerns over having her as a passenger.

Many moms conjure up an invisible foot brake when their teenage offspring are behind the wheel. Almost every mother I've known, from childhood to my now fortysomething friends, possesses a primal instinct that causes them to fling their arm bolt straight from their body to protect their passenger—of any age—from the impact of a short stop. I have a theory that it's the human chorionic gonadotropin secreted during pregnancy, because I don't do it, myself, but science may never know.

What I do know is that on the homebound leg of that particular journey, Mumsie, a nervous passenger on her calmest days, was stomping the ghost brake, flailing and gasping as I piloted the Slutmobile through late rush-hour traffic. As she braced in anticipation of a semitricky left-hand merge onto I-75, I was attempting to breathe as deeply as I could to ward off her worry, which was also beginning to merge with my own. Spying an opening in the traffic, I floored it, needing the momentum to propel the car across four lanes of fast-moving vehicles to our exit on the right. But when I gunned it, the engine ground. We were drifting and slowing, horns blaring all around us as the traffic around us split and swarmed. Mumsie threw her hands over her eyes and I envied her that respite, swiveling my head around to determine the cause of our sudden halt. And there it was: her thrashing hand had knocked the gearshift into neutral.

I cursed, loudly and profanely, and once we were parked I vowed two things: that I would never allow her to take that drive with me again, and that I'd never, ever be the nervous passenger.

I've kept one of them.

It came on all of a sudden during my honeymoon. We'd rented a small, sporty car that the hotel concierge assured my brandnew groom would be well suited to the hairpin, single-track roads between London and the tiny Welsh town where a friend had gotten us a cottage for the week. All was going swimmingly until it was time to leave the city, and I'll say this in my defense: London traffic sucks. There is no circumnavigating the fact that it's a nasty snarl of too many taxis, buses, and lorries, copious roundabouts, and civilian drivers—freed of British politesse by the boundary of a windshield— angry at the world for all of the above. It's tense and terrible, but Douglas was handling it with great aplomb. I, on the other hand, was a mental wreck. I had yet to come down from the adrenaline overload of our wedding and the aftermath, as we'd rushed from wrapping up the festivities, driving back to the city, kenneling the dogs, packing, and getting to the airport for a red-eye transatlantic flight that very night. A light breeze could have set me on edge. In this case, it was other vehicles, then low, stone walls and precipitous cliff drops coming at me from an up-close angle and a side I wasn't used to. I've been to the UK plenty of times, but had done almost all my travel by tube or foot, and the low set of the car set me on edge in a way I could never have expected. Where we were going, there was no option but to drive on cramped, cobbled, sheep-strewn roads while I held my breath and crunched my shoulders inward as if narrowing the outline of my body would somehow keep the car from scraping against brambles and bumpers or plummeting over too-close edges. When I'd vowed not to part from him till death, I hadn't anticipated such a thing coming within the next week.

We'd spent money on the wedding—technically less than the national average (it helps when your husband-to-be owns an actual church building), but still more than pocket change. My most recent freelance job had just ended and the second we left on our honeymoon, Douglas's rotten, stinking, no-good business partner had drained almost all the cash from their company's accounts. Castles, naps, and special grown-up-married-people time was bookended by jaunts to the local library to check e-mail to make sure that his employees hadn't set the offices ablaze and sold the copy machines for scrap. Every bump in the road and hairpin turn felt like cash jangling out of our pockets and I couldn't stop from flinching. Why hadn't we opted for a Smart car or a battered old Citroën? This fancy thing was going to get wrecked, or we'd smash into something and have to pay money we increasingly didn't have.

Along with the commemorative Snowdonian castle map tea towels and snapshots of ourselves amid various ruins, crags, and sheep, I brought back with me from that trip a fear of sitting in the passenger's seat of a car for which I have financial responsibility. Could be a rental, could be my very own Chrysler (which I have driven only once, by the way—once, while Douglas hauls my trembling carcass around), but the on switch got flipped and I have yet to change the station.

Mumsie had an excuse: a learned fearfulness from her father, who'd seen his uncle badly injured in a car accident, and it trickled down to me. I could cling to that as a justification for why I flinch and gasp when we drift slightly toward the boundaries of our lane, inch almost imperceptibly closer to the car in front of us—the car I am sure will suddenly brake and not all the flung-out arms in the world will save us from destroying—or why I press my hand to the roof to brace when we whiz between a guardrail and a sky-blocking Mack truck. Someday I'll grab the wheel—maybe at the next stop.

Closing Scene

I wish I could lie to you, tell you that I figured out a magical way not to worry, and that *poof* it'll work for you, too. I wish I could claim that some specific mantra, posture, diet, app, guru, or pill sieved the upset from me, and after all this, I'm about to whisper it in your ear and fix you. Lean closer.

I'm sorry, but I can't. I would if I could. But I'm not ashamed—and that's what's changed.

When I came out as anxious in a widely read essay at the beginning of 2014, the protective bubble I'd carefully crafted for myself smashed open. I was the one swinging the hammer. I had to. You can suffocate in your own shame over things that are simply a part of you. Fine if it's just me, freak of nature that I am, who gets palpitations at the notion of leaving the house to walk down the block to get half-and-half, and would rather let penalty fees accrue than pick up the phone and talk to another person about how I'd failed at the basic business of being an adult. Fine. But my illness was starting to infect and injure people I love and I just couldn't live with that.

Your friend doesn't show up for your party once: okay. They were sick, maybe overscheduled, life happens. But then they don't get in touch for months, don't return your e-mails and texts, duck making plans, yet seem to be perfectly alive and well on the Internet. You can chalk it up to their being a thoughtless jerk, and that might be the case. Or you might wonder what's wrong with you, if you completely misjudged your worth to them and the level of friendship you thought you'd shared. You might be angry with them, worried for them, or turn it in on yourself, deeply wounded by the loss and second-guessing every conversation you'd shared.

That winter, after too many skipped holiday parties, bailed-on drinks, panic attacks in public places, and texts from friends asking if it was something they said, I came clean. I'm sick, and this is an explanation, not an excuse. I've been this way all along, I've tried everything to fight it, I've tried to hide it from you. I hope you don't stop loving me now that you know.

It was the most terrifying thing I'd ever done, scrubbing down to bare skin and striding into the spotlight, and also the most liberating. It's exhausting, trying to masquerade as a well person when you're not one. The things that most people take for granted—being able to leave the house, go to work, hold down a job even, pick up the phone, go on a date, see a friend, drive a car, pay a bill—take so much extra effort when there's an iron vise keeping you from breathing. Having to pretend for everyone else's sake that you're okay so they keep liking, respecting, trusting, or employing you, or to spare them the worry—it's a full-time job. I had to take the risk and quit that job or it was going to kill me.

I realized quickly that I was privileged as hell in a way that many people who suffer from mental illness aren't. I've got a partner who also works, health insurance and access to care, a grad school education, friends and family who freely talk about mental health issues and see them on par with the physical, no religious restrictions, no major physical impediments, and most crucially in this case, an employer who was on board with the whole revelation. Not only was I not penalized at work for coming clean, they made it front-page news, let me host an online chat with experts, and encouraged me to keep the conversation going.

This is not the norm; far from it, in fact. While I was buoyed up by the unexpected support of thousands of people, friends and strangers, telling me that I was not unlovable or alone, so many others came to me whispering: I can tell you because you won't judge me, but my partner, my church, my culture, my family, my boss—they can never know. They'll think I'm crazy. They say I should just put my faith in God. We just don't talk about it. I don't want to worry them. They'll think I'm weak and messed up and should tough it out. I'll lose my job. They won't understand. And even if they did, I don't have the money for treatment or medication. And if I had that, there is no one around here to go to. I'd have to go to another town, and that scares me, I can't afford it, I can't physically manage it, I can't take the time away. I think I'll always be this way.

This bothers me more than anything—the thought that people are suffering, and it's compounded because of a cruel taboo. Through all the therapy, medication, mind and body exercises, meditation, and countless methods I've tried, absolutely nothing has helped as much as simply being able to talk about my anxiety. To have the freedom to say that I'm not okay and that I don't have to apologize for it. I have plenty of work to do on myself and I've accepted the fact that I may never be fully "cured" of my anxiety. Knowing that there are good, smart, lovable people who share my struggles has made all of the difference in the world to me. I'm not alone and we're not broken.

I've met people of every age, race, skin color, religion, gender, sexuality, income and education level who have told me that they grapple with anxiety every day, and that a large part of the burden comes from having to hide it from the people around them. Considering that 18 percent of the U.S.'s adult population has been diagnosed with some form of anxiety-related mental condition, there's an awfully good chance that if I'm in a room with five other people, at least one of them struggled to wake up and put on their Calm Person suit that day. That's just the people who have been diagnosed and managed to leave the house—and I'd probably never guess which ones they are. Anxiety is usually invisible.

This is not just nervousness. This is not some silly fretting that can be snapped out of. This is not weakness. This is not craziness. This is not anything to be ashamed of. But this illness is hurting someone you love, and robbing them of the life and joy they deserve—not to mention the care. We should want better for them. And ourselves.

That's why I wrote this book, even though it often felt like scraping off my skin with a butter knife. For as terrible as it feels to live in my body some days, it's gotten infinitely easier since I allowed myself to live in the open. And I'm pretty much not going to shut up about this until everyone else has that freedom, too. I'm not suggesting some sort of mandatory annual national wellness retreat where we all schlep out to the desert with yoga mats and Nalgene bottles full of weird-smelling sixteen-dollar "calming" teas to commune with our inner wind puppet. I'm sure that's marvelous and healing for some people, but prohibitively costly and time-consuming for most. It also may or may not work: just like mindfulness, yoga, apps, chants, prayers, supplements, prescriptions, exercise, or any given therapy technique might be the key to your personal calm, or might add to your agitation.

But doing nothing and staying quiet isn't an option either. Not for me. I have to believe that if I yell loudly enough, other voices will join in. And once there are too many of us to be ignored, we won't be afraid to demand the compassion we deserve.

'm squirming in my airplane seat all the way home. Douglas lost his mother a week and a half before, after a good, long life with a sharp downward drift at the end. Work took me away for a few days and I was aching to get back to him and home, but when I come through the door, something just isn't quite right. Something different from the soft-edged, familiar sadness that had blanketed our apartment since she'd started to descend.

Sit down, he tells me, and my chest ices over. There's no easy way to tell you, so I'll just come out with it. Your dad sent me an e-mail, he didn't seem to want to talk on the phone. Your mom has declined so much she'll have to be moved into a nursing home or a hospice. They think she has a year. Maybe two. And he can't handle her care anymore because he'll be starting cancer treatment and he'll need all his strength. I'm so sorry to have to tell you this.

For once, I do not worry. I am beyond that. Not just because shortly after that, I ask Douglas to walk with me to a bar and I pour gin on my nerves until they drown, but because worrying will not help. This is happening, and once the numb of this night wears off, I do not have the luxury or impediment of feeling—only doing, helping, being useful. I set my jaw.

Soon after, I am driving hours through thunder unafraid, surprising them at their door. Pup seems tired, but himself, and happy I'm there. Her mouth drops open and stays that way long enough for me to be sure that she knows who I am. How could she not? I think. We look like ghosts of each other. A few weeks later, I am in an avalanche of Bubble Wrap, swaddling the sharp edges of books, paintings, pictures of the life they had together. Mumsie has already been moved from their retirement home to a nursing home and Pup will be living with my sister to preserve his strength and cash. His treatment is working well, he tells me. He seems at peace with what is going on inside his bones, but fusses worriedly when I am several minutes late, reminds me which curves are blind and intersections are tricky. I have to laugh. I fret just as much when Douglas is on the road or in the air out of my sight. No need to wrap up any tchotchkes and nestle them in my luggage—I already have my inheritance.

We ready ourselves to go over and see Mumsie. It's only been a few weeks since I've seen her, but he wants me to be prepared for how much she has declined in that time. The TIAs had eroded her brain, but a nasty, messy brew of Alzheimer's, Parkinson's, and Lewy body dementia has welled up to draw her under. In those weeks, she has lost the ability to shuffle from recliner to couch with her walker. She is confined to a wheelchair. She chokes on her food and has required the Heimlich twice since moving in, so her meals are now pureed. I turn around for a moment and gasp in pain when I hear that, but wheel back, all smiles, when I stride through the door toward the activities area. There are whole walnuts on the table and no one seems to know or care quite why, but Mumsie's face tightens slightly from listless to shocked when I walk up to her. Pleasure seems just out of her range of expression, but I hear my name come from her mouth for the first time in years and it feels as fierce as a hug. Pup wheels her to her room—neat and warm and studded with familiar objects from home. I sit in a chair facing her. The disease is attempting to draw her into herself and her chin tips forward to meet her breastbone. Though it's hard for her to find and form words, it seems she's struggling to listen. The way the diseases have ravaged her brain, it's hard for her to form new memories, so I try to marry what I'm saying to things I know . . . and I hope are etched bone-deep. Remember that little girl with cancer you used to send cards to? She's grown up now, just had a baby of her own. Remember my friend who used to come over and sing while I played the piano? She's the principal of the school where we met in kindergarten. Remember how I always used to scribble those little poems and stories? I'm writing a book now. Remember my husband, Douglas? He makes me feel safe and loved every day.

She's fading and it seems almost cruel to keep her awake, but there is still so much I want her to know. It's time, though, and Pup gently pleads with her to try and remember that the movers are coming tomorrow, so he might not come by. Please don't panic and have the staff call because you are convinced I am dead on the road. Please try. She was better about this for a while, he tells me. She learned some wonderful techniques for coping with panic in group therapy after she broke down, but she just doesn't have the cognitive function to employ them anymore. When Pup and I are getting our coats, she frets, afraid we're leaving her behind in her room. Who will take her to lunch? We've got you, we promise. We'll take care of you.

There's a little bit of time before I have to leave and I spend it with Pup. Of course I'm a little bit antsy about returning my rental car, catching my flight, but I tamp that down as best I can. He is here, solid and in the flesh, and that is so much more important than the specter of some minor, solvable problem that may or may not come to pass. I'll come back soon. I know you will take care of her. Please take care of yourself.

And then I'm back on a plane headed home. It's not a crowded flight and I'm randomly upgraded to first class, so I can let my body still and sprawl. It's a minor luxury before I crash-land back into my real life, so I take a deep breath, hold it in, and do my best to fly above it all.

I'm Kat. I'm my Mumsie's daughter. Anxiety is not the only thing that ties us together.

ACKNOWLEDGMENTS

Shockingly enough, I have been incredibly nervous about writing these acknowledgments for fear that I'd leave out someone important and then they'd hate me and the world would end. But here we go.

Thank you, Carrie Thornton, my editor and friend, for being both of those things. You were the one who told me I should write this book, and you made feel safe and supported enough to dig deeply, painfully at some times, so I could write an honest book we could both be proud of. IOU many dinners at the Nep. Eric and John, I wish you could be there with us.

Thank you, Sean Newcott, Lauren Janiec, and Tanya Leet from HarperCollins for shepherding a first-time author through this crazy process with humor and patience. Thank you as well to Julie Paulauski, Lynn Grady, Michael Barrs, and Stephanie Vallejo.

Thank you, Scott Mendel, for being the absolutely perfect agent for an anxious writer. Your grace, humor, and kindness are so deeply appreciated.

Thank you, Melonyce McAfee and Jamie Gumbrecht, for holding my hand through those CNN essays. Without your editorial guidance and open hearts, none of this would have happened.

Thank you, Meredith Artley, K. C. Estenson, Manuel Perez, Mira Lowe, and Susan Grant for creating a workplace that encouraged boldness and creativity, and for letting me use CNN.com as a platform to have a national conversation about mental illness. I know what a rare, risky thing that is, and I am so lucky to have worked there.

Thank you, Jen Doll, for the long lunch that gave me the kick in the ass I needed to move forward.

Thank you, Jennifer V. Cole, Pete Wells, Bill Addison, and Helen Rosner for being just a text away when I was writing and feeling utterly batshit.

Thank you, Bridget Mora, Alison Dorfman, and Sarah LeTrent for being my girls, always.

Thank you, Pamela McQueen, Lissa Townsend Rodgers, Sean Elder, and Steven Stern for telling me early on that I should maybe possibly think about giving writing a chance.

Thank you, Susan Merwin, Benjamin Fialkoff, Peter Wildeman, Victoria Albina, and Terry Cramer for taking good, kind care of my brain throughout the years. That is not a tiny job.

Thank you, Elissa Schappell, Bret Thorne, Robert Sorkin, and Adair Iacono for each seeing me in a vulnerable moment and not judging.

Thank you, Josh Ozersky, for making me unafraid to dance without apology. And thank you, Sarah Abell, for dancing with me.

Thank you, Geoff Bartakovics and Kai Mathey, for being flexible so I could tackle this beast.

Thank you, Rainbow Rowell, Beach House, The xx and Washed Out for making the art I had on repeat while I was writing this book. It put my brain and my soul in the right place.

Thank you, Jaya Miceli, for absolutely nailing the cover design on the first try.

Thank you, Chadwick Boyd, Phil Baltz, Stacey Ballis and Martha Martin for the surprise pep talks that made me believe that the world would give a damn about what I had to say.

Thank you, Dana Cowin and Dorothy Kalins for your mentorship, kindness, and guidance. You are my role models in work and in life.

Thank you, Nan and Polly for stepping in when I didn't know how to ask.

Thank you, Mumsie and Pup, for showing me what lifelong love can look like, being my creative champions, giving me the space to be a complete weirdo, helping me find the language to talk about how I was feeling, and for getting me care so early on. I am grateful for you every day.

Thank you, Douglas, for being my home, my love, and my north. This book is my love letter to you.

And thank you to every thoughful, generous person who opened up your heart to me along the way—in person, in e-mails, in comments, on Facebook and Twitter—to say, "Me, too." Even if we never meet, you have made my life better, I have felt so much less alone because of your words and actions, and I will always be grateful.

ABOUT THE AUTHOR

Kat Kinsman is the senior food and drinks editor for Time Inc.'s all-breakfast website Extra Crispy and founder of Chefs With Issues, a website dedicated to raising awareness about mental health issues in the food world. She is the former editor in chief and editor at large of *Tasting Table*. She was the founding editor of CNN's Eatocracy, edited CNN's matrimony section, First Person essay series, and wrote for CNN Living. She has been nominated for the James Beard Broadcast Award in the TV Segment category and won the 2011 EPPY Best Food Website. A former senior editor for AOL Food and Slashfood, she was a longtime member of the James Beard Journalism Committee, does frequent public speaking on food and mental health issues, and has appeared on CNN, HLN TV, CNN Radio, and *Good Morning America*. She lives in Brooklyn, New York, with her husband, Douglas, and various animals.